GET STRONG

FOR WOMEN

LIFT HEAVY ⬤ TRAIN HARD ⬤ SEE RESULTS

ALEX SILVER-FAGAN

CONTENTS

LOWER BODY

POWER

THE PROGRAMMES

LEVEL 1

LEVEL 2

LEVEL 3

INTRODUCTION

Even though more women strength train now than ever before, there is still a myth floating around that lifting weights will make women bulky. As for the women who already strength train, the majority of them simply aren't training properly or with enough resistance to produce an effect.

One thing we can all agree on, however, is that as women we want to feel strong, empowered, and confident. So, I'm here to dispel the myths you hear and to help you achieve true strength in and out of the gym.

This book is for you – to help you reap the benefits of lifting weights the right way. *Get Strong for Women* will help you train with the proper exercises and with the proper intensity. This book will help you train with confidence.

Lifting weights will make you stronger, healthier, and leaner, but the benefits go beyond just the physical. Strength training improves your confidence, lessens your stress levels, and helps you develop overall mental toughness.

How do I know? Because I have watched my own body and my own life change, along with the lives of my clients, by using a smart and systematic training programme. As a personal trainer, certified strength coach, and group fitness instructor, I have worked with clients of all different levels and ages, helping them to get fit, healthy, strong, and capable of anything.

With 61 exercises and three 12-week programmes based on your fitness level, this book provides all the information and tips you need to GET STRONG, regardless of your goals or your starting point.

So let's do this.
Let's get strong together.

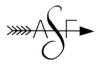

ALEX SILVER-FAGAN

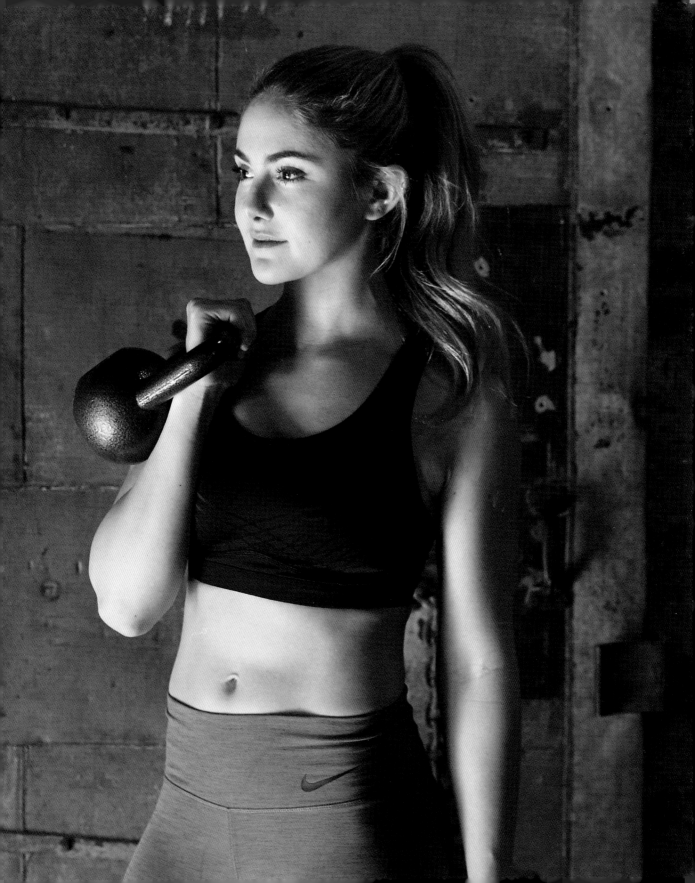

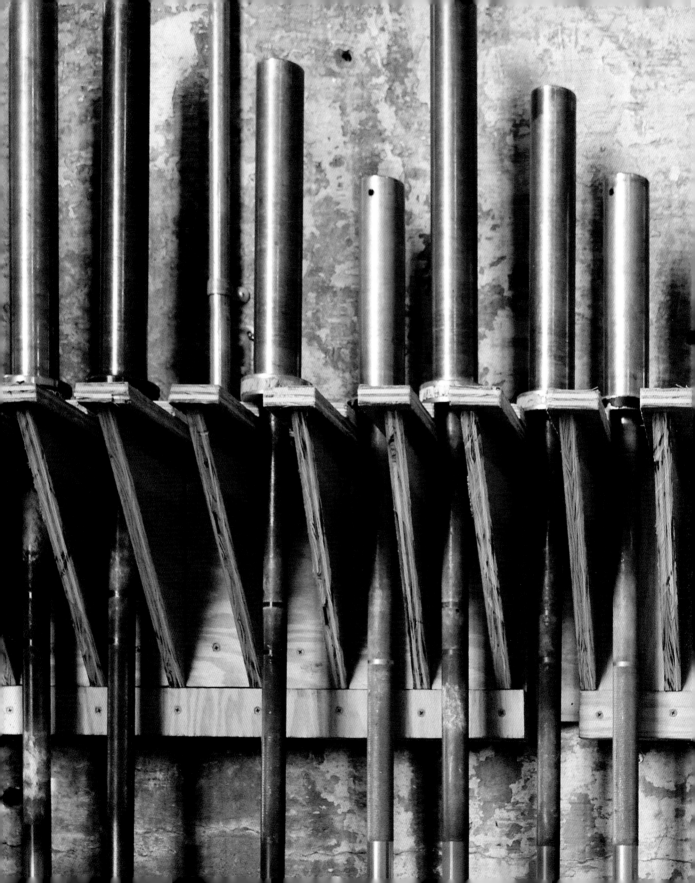

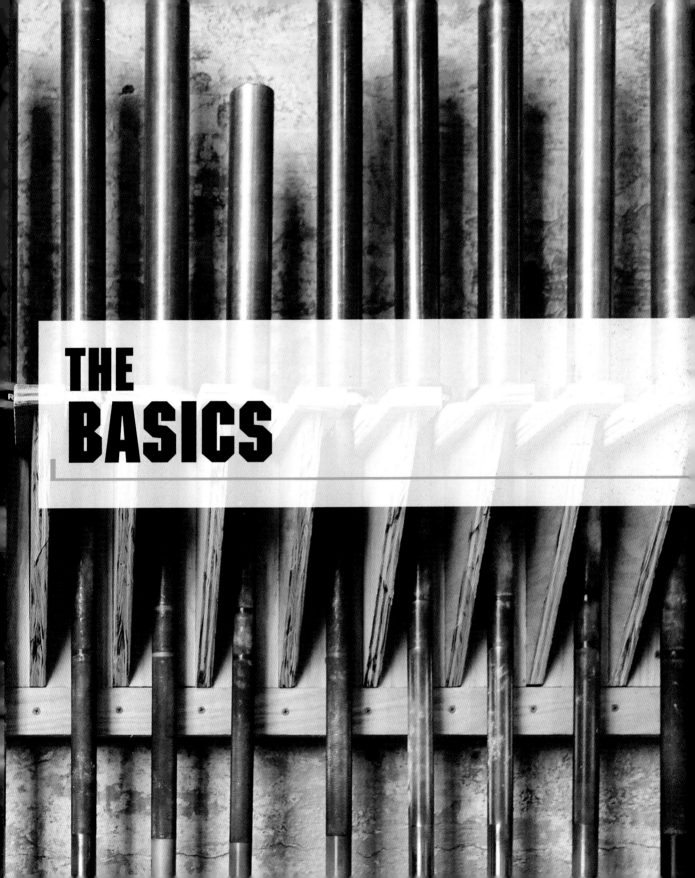

THE
BASICS

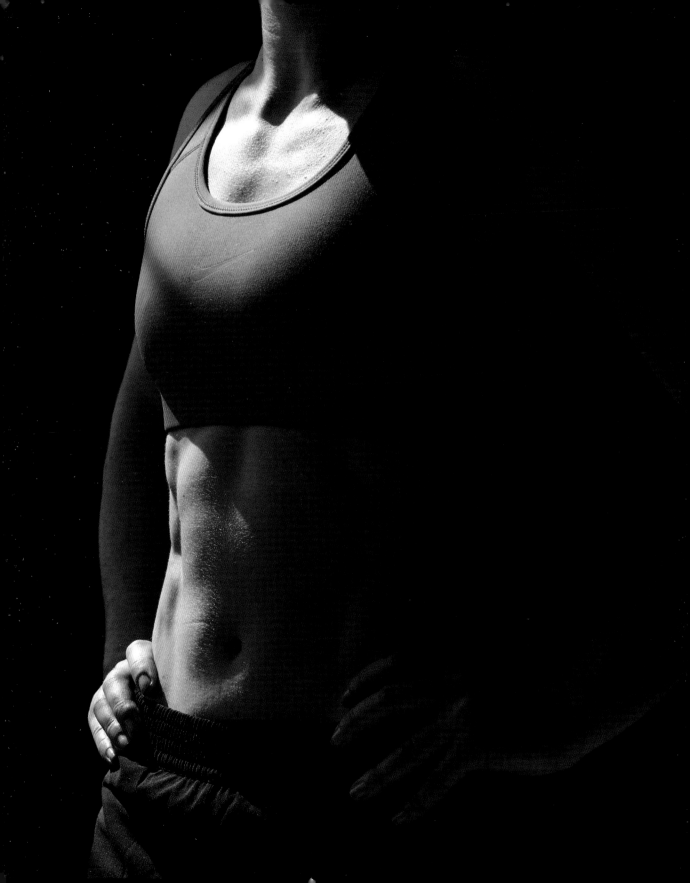

WHY GET STRONG?

The best way to sculpt a healthy physique is by training with resistance, and with proper training, your body is capable of lifting very heavy weights. The movements you do in the weights room translate to stronger, more confident movements in your daily life, empowering both your body and your mind.

BUILD CONFIDENCE

You'll be surprised by how quickly the shape of your body begins to change when you lift heavy weights. Even within the first week, your muscles will feel firmer and more defined. Plus, when you work out, your body releases endorphins, chemicals produced in the brain that can boost your mood and relax you during times of stress or pain. Exercising triggers actual positive feelings. Your resulting confidence and euphoria are not superficial – they are your body's natural way of encouraging healthy fitness, which rewards you with a more sculpted body and more graceful movement.

ENHANCE LEAN MUSCLE MASS

Lifting weights and training for power will increase your body's lean muscle mass. Do not let the fear of getting big or bulky dissuade you from heavy lifting. In reality, the opposite is true; although muscle weighs more than fat, it occupies less space and is more shapely. Even though you might not see the number on the scales go down as you gain muscle mass, you will notice a drastic difference in your appearance as you become slimmer and more sculpted. Your glutes will become tighter, your waist trimmer, your legs leaner, and your posture taller and stronger.

IMPROVE FUNCTIONAL MOVEMENT

By training your body in multiple planes of motion with added resistance, you also improve the way you move in daily life. The movement patterns you execute in the weights room translate to more stable, flexible, and balanced movement in general – no matter where you are. This functional training approach reduces your risk of injury and lets you confidently approach any movement challenge.

REDUCE BODY FAT

Strength training causes a lot of stress on your body – in a good way. This extra resistance forces the body to work hard to recover, which heightens your metabolism while at the same time increasing muscle mass. Lifting weights boosts your resting metabolic rate (also known as your RMR), meaning that you will burn more calories throughout the day, even long after you've left the gym.

> " Taking control of your **strength** means taking control of your life. You will be more **confident** in your body, its capabilities, and your own **discipline**. "

BUILDING STRENGTH

Getting strong doesn't happen overnight. It is a gradual process that requires commitment to routine, dedication to form, and drive to continually push yourself every day. Each time you pick up a weight, you are training your muscles to become stronger and more adept at functional movement.

PUSH YOUR MUSCLES

Your body adapts to the type of work you demand of it. If you habitually lift heavy weights, your body responds by building the muscular strength and power to support the activity. That's how strength training works – you overload your muscles, allow them to adapt, then overload again.

An effective training programme is one that keeps your body guessing by varying the movements and challenging your body with greater resistance. This way, your body never gets comfortable, and your progress never halts. The programmes in this book will pull your body out of that comfort zone so that you see results.

BUILD MUSCLE MASS

On a microscopic level, resistance training builds your skeletal muscle mass – the muscles attached to bones and tendons that are responsible for the force behind all your movement. These muscles are composed of individual muscle fibres. When your muscles work against external resistance, such as when lifting weights, this causes microscopic tears in your muscle fibres.

After your workout, your body repairs these damaged fibres, making them stronger and thicker than before. As you continue to train, your muscles grow in size and definition. Gradually increasing the amount of weight you lift ensures that your muscles continue to build.

MOVE FUNCTIONALLY

Building strength should not mean that you become muscle-bound or lose flexibility. A strong body is one that is able to move fluidly. For this reason, the movements in the book are functional, meaning they challenge your body to move as it is naturally designed to: in multiple planes of motion and in fluid, compound movements.

Effective functional strength training employs the seven foundational movement patterns: squat, lunge, push, pull, hinge, twist, and walk. Together, these patterns of movement occupy all planes of motion and keep your body healthy and injury-free.

" If you want to **get strong**, you have to **train hard**. Push your muscles and monitor your progress. You will **see results**. "

WHAT NEXT?

You probably have lots of questions about getting started. These are a few of the most common concerns women have when they begin strength training.

Q Do women need to train differently to men?

A Women and men have different hormonal profiles, which affects how muscle is gained. Because we have less testosterone, our bodies don't physically build muscle mass in the same way that men's bodies do. However, the training principles that build strength in men are equally effective for building strength in women.

Q When will I start to see results?

A Everyone responds differently to training. Physically, you may start to feel a little stronger and more fit within the first four weeks of training. Mentally, you will feel more confident as soon as you start a programme. Don't rely on the scales as your only measure of progress. When you lift weights, you'll be adding lean muscle mass, which means your weight may go up, but your body fat will go down, and you will look leaner and fitter.

Q Isn't cardio better for boosting my metabolism and making me look lean?

A Cardio is important for boosting your metabolism and shedding fat, but it is not better than weight training. In order to build the body you want and to be as fit as possible, you need a mix of both weight training and cardio. The programmes in this book emphasize weight training to build muscle and increase your metabolism, but also include cardio finishers at the end of the workouts to raise your heart rate. Ultimately, cardio is important for your overall health, as it improves cardiovascular performance and endurance.

Q What causes muscle soreness? What if I don't get sore after a workout?

A Muscle soreness is caused by the microscopic tears created in the muscle fibres during exercise (not the build-up of lactic acid, as many believe). This

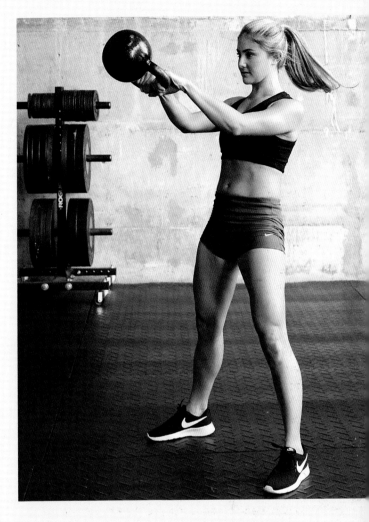

damage results in soreness and pain. Swelling occurs along with soreness, so your muscles may look puffy and larger than before.

If you don't feel sore after a workout, it's either because you didn't overload your muscles, or because you've been working hard for an extended period of time and your muscles have acclimatized to the stress. If you're just starting out and not getting sore, consider increasing your resistance. If you've been working out for a while, consider increasing weight or decreasing rest time.

However, don't let muscle soreness be the only indicator of a good training session. It's more important to know your limits, push past them just a little bit, eat well, and recover!

NUTRITION FOR YOUR BODY

Strength training is most effective when you feed your body the right balance of basic nutrients. This requires eating with awareness and, at first, tracking what you eat so that you can see the nutrient breakdown of your current diet and make adjustments as needed. Remember that your body needs fuel, so don't cut calories drastically.

BASIC NUTRIENTS

The best way to eat strategically is to understand the macronutrients (macros) in your diet. These are the caloric building blocks of food: carbohydrates, protein, and fat. Each macro provides you with unique benefits, and understanding the macro composition of your diet helps you control how your body looks and moves. While macro tracking shouldn't be a lifelong goal, it's a helpful tool when beginning your journey. If you regulate the ratio of the three macros in your diet for a while, you can find a ratio that keeps you lean and helps you gain muscle. The easiest way to track diet is with a fitness app such as *MyFitnessPal* or *My Macros+*.

CARBOHYDRATES

Energy
4 calories/gram

Function
Carbohydrates are your primary energy source and incredibly important when training. It's best to focus on complex carbohydrates (found in vegetables and whole grains), which digest slowly for efficient vitamin and mineral intake, and keep you fuller for longer. Simple carbohydrates (found in fruits, milk, and sugar) digest quickly and are helpful for a quick burst of energy, but can also contribute to unnecessary body fat.

Best sources
Whole grains, green vegetables, starchy vegetables, legumes

PROTEIN

Energy
4 calories/gram

Function
Protein is a combination of amino acids that stimulate recovery and muscle growth in the body. This macro is necessary for your cells to function, grow, and properly regulate your body's tissues and organs. Getting an adequate amount of protein is non-negotiable, whether you are training or not. For most people, protein should make up the bulk of your meals.

Best sources
Meat, seafood, dairy products, eggs, legumes, soya

FAT

Energy
9 calories/gram

Function
Fat is an essential nutrient for many bodily functions. It's crucial for cell communication throughout the body, and also helps to absorb vitamins and promote hormone secretion. It is a very dense macronutrient, which means a small portion is high in calories but also keeps you full. Don't avoid foods that are high in fat, but seek out those that deliver other benefits as well, such as high protein content or a high concentration of omega-3s.

Best sources
Avocados, salmon, nuts, olive oil, coconut

DIFFERENT BODIES, DIFFERENT DIETS

While each person's body is unique, most people can generally categorize themselves into one of three types of body compositions: ectomorph, mesomorph, and endomorph. Knowing your type helps you understand the best macro ratio for your body. These types are not just related to physique, but they also respond to and process macronutrients differently.

ECTOMORPH

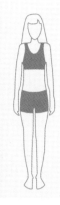

Ectomorph body type
- Tall stature
- Smaller bone structure
- High metabolism
- Gain and lose fat slowly
- Gain and lose muscle slowly

Ideal macro breakdown

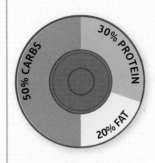

50% CARBS · 30% PROTEIN · 20% FAT

Meal planning
Ectomorphs need a higher ratio of carbs to fat. Each meal should include:
- 1 palm-sized serving of protein
- 1 fist-sized serving of vegetables
- 2 handfuls of whole grains or legumes
- ½ thumb-sized portion of fat

MESOMORPH

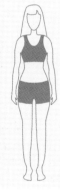

Mesomorph body type
- Rectangular-shaped body
- Athletic build
- Gain and lose fat easily
- Gain and lose muscle easily

Ideal macro breakdown

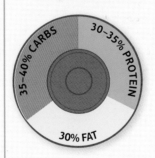

35–40% CARBS · 30–35% PROTEIN · 30% FAT

Meal planning
Mesomorphs require a balanced macro ratio, with lower carbs if trying to lose weight. Each meal should include:
- 1 palm-sized serving of protein
- 1 fist-sized serving of vegetables
- 1 handful of whole grains or legumes
- 1 thumb-sized portion of fat

ENDOMORPH

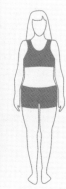

Endomorph body type
- Stocky or round physique
- Broad bone structure
- Gain fat and muscle easily
- Lose fat slowly

Ideal macro breakdown

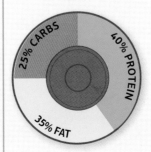

25% CARBS · 40% PROTEIN · 35% FAT

Meal planning
Endomorphs need a lower ratio of carbs to fat. Each meal should include:
- 1 palm-sized serving of protein
- 1 fist-sized serving of vegetables
- ½ handful of whole grains or legumes
- 2 thumb-sized portions of fat

NUTRITION WHEN TRAINING

Your body requires energy to support a good workout and the right foods to build muscle mass. Eating nutrient-dense, healthy meals when hungry will help you feel well all day long and encourage quick results. Dietary supplements may also help you reach your goals efficiently.

STAYING HYDRATED

Drinking enough water is the key to effective training and good health. Your body is composed of 80 per cent water, and it plays a vital role in nearly every bodily function. It helps transport and metabolize nutrients for good digestion, as well as removing toxins from your body. Stay hydrated by drinking at least eight 240ml (8fl oz) glasses of water per day.

FOODS TO AVOID

If your goal is to build strength and lose fat, then processed foods and sugar (packaged foods and desserts) should not find their way onto your plate. Your body turns these simple carbs into stored fat without gaining any nutrients. Cutting out or cutting down on alcohol is another great fat loss tool – alcohol is a simple sugar and provides no nutrition.

BEFORE AND AFTER TRAINING

This book won't tell you exactly when to eat and work out, but you can follow the guidelines below to make sure your body is adequately fuelled. Rely on full, balanced meals when you are hungry, and fill in with snacks to accommodate your fitness schedule. For example, if you work out early in the morning, eat a banana before, and eat a complete breakfast for your post-workout nutrition.

BEFORE

To power your workout, it is important to eat a balanced meal two to three hours beforehand. Training on an empty stomach causes your body to burn protein from your muscles for energy instead of glucose sugars (from carbohydrates) found in your kidneys and liver. If you need a snack just before a training session, complex carbs and protein are best. However, you should avoid fatty foods and overeating just before, which can cause indigestion and sluggishness.

Pre-workout snacks
▶ Banana and nut butter
▶ Apple and nuts
▶ Porridge with berries
▶ Rice cake with nut butter

AFTER

Following a workout, your muscles crave energy to repair the fibres and build more mass. To fuel your recovery, eat a full meal that includes protein and complex carbs within 30 minutes of your workout. Consuming fat right away might slow the absorption of nutrients from your meal, but it won't reduce its benefits or harm you.

Post-workout meals
▶ Wholemeal wrap with turkey and vegetables
▶ Grilled chicken and sweet potato
▶ Egg-white omelette with vegetables
▶ Protein shake (protein powder with either water or almond milk)

WHAT ABOUT SUPPLEMENTS?

You should always rely primarily on whole foods to provide your body with the nutrition and vitamins that it needs, and use supplements as a secondary tool. The following may balance your nutrition and help you reach your goals:

▶ **Protein powder** For the average busy woman, getting enough protein can be difficult. Protein shakes are one way to ensure you get the proper amount of protein to recover and rebuild your muscles. Powders come from many different sources (whey, casein, egg, plant, etc) to suit your dietary preferences.

▶ **BCAAs** Short for branched-chain amino acids, these supplements can take your muscle growth to the next level. BCAAs are the building blocks of muscle and help speed up protein synthesis, which will improve post-workout recovery. They can be taken during a workout or after, or even throughout the day. BCAAs are a great alternative to sugary sports drinks.

▶ **Fish oil** A fish oil supplement, which is rich in omega-3, reduces inflammation in the body. It provides essential fatty acids such as EPA and DHA, which play key roles in cognitive health and development.

▶ **Multivitamin** A basic multivitamin provides a long list of necessary vitamins and nutrients that your body may not be getting from your diet.

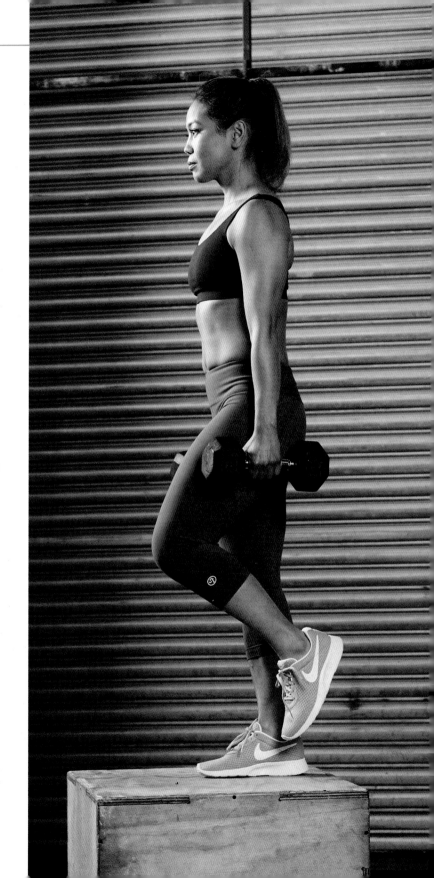

EQUIPMENT

The exercises in this book use a variety of equipment to help you overload your muscles and produce results. You may find a setup similar to this at your gym.

Pull-up bar
This is a fixed horizontal bar that's often attached to the top of a power rack, or sometimes freestanding. You can hang on it for pull-ups and chin-ups.

Rings or TRX
Gymnastic rings or a suspension training system (TRX) are used for the same exercises. You hold on to suspended rings or handles to perform total-body pushing and pulling exercises. Resistance can be increased or decreased based on your body's angle to the floor.

Power rack
This large structure has adjustable hooks on the sides, which let you set a barbell at custom heights. You can also attach safety bars to the rack so that you can lift without a spotter.

Plyo boxes
Short for plyometric, these boxes are used for jumping and stepping exercises. They vary in height and come in both wood and soft foam.

Clips
These secure the weight plates to the bar.

Medicine balls
Cushioned and filled with sand, these balls range in weight from 1 to 12 kilograms.

Dumbbells
These are like mini barbells. You hold them freely in one hand, and they're great for isolation exercises. Weights range from 0.5 to 50 kilograms and up.

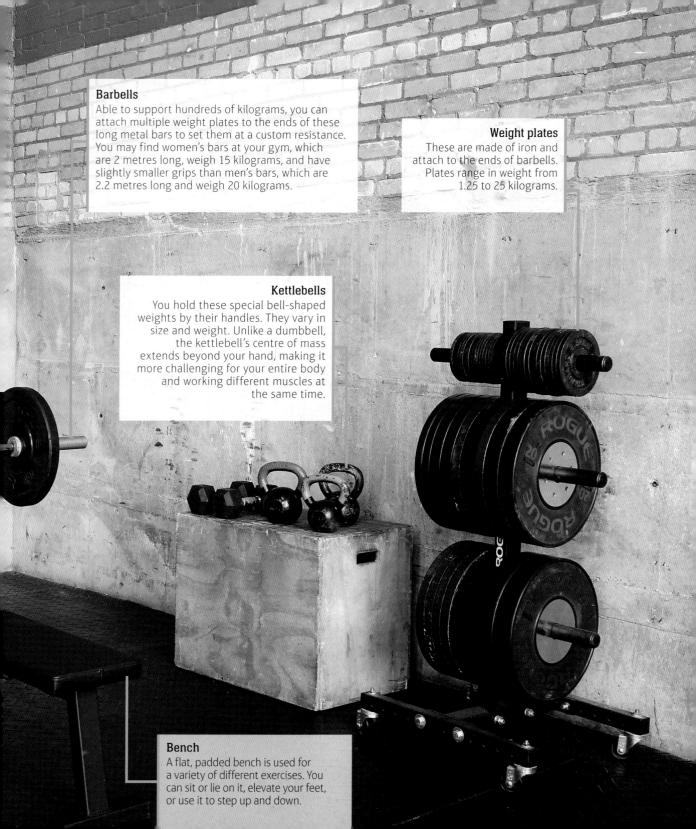

Barbells
Able to support hundreds of kilograms, you can attach multiple weight plates to the ends of these long metal bars to set them at a custom resistance. You may find women's bars at your gym, which are 2 metres long, weigh 15 kilograms, and have slightly smaller grips than men's bars, which are 2.2 metres long and weigh 20 kilograms.

Weight plates
These are made of iron and attach to the ends of barbells. Plates range in weight from 1.25 to 25 kilograms.

Kettlebells
You hold these special bell-shaped weights by their handles. They vary in size and weight. Unlike a dumbbell, the kettlebell's centre of mass extends beyond your hand, making it more challenging for your entire body and working different muscles at the same time.

Bench
A flat, padded bench is used for a variety of different exercises. You can sit or lie on it, elevate your feet, or use it to step up and down.

GETTING STARTED

Before you head into the weights room, you need to select a training programme to keep you safe and accountable. There are three 12-week programmes in this book, designed for a range of abilities. Complete the simple fitness assessment below to help you pick the level that's most suitable for you.

ASSESS YOUR FITNESS

Before beginning your 12-week *Get Strong* programme, use this timed bodyweight test to assess your current strength and endurance. The results tell you which of the three programme levels to follow.

TIME YOURSELF

Perform the exercises back to back as quickly as you can for the specified number of reps. Use a stopwatch to record how long it takes you to complete the sequence. Don't stop the timer until you've completed the last 5 burpees.

► 15 push-ups

► 15 squats

► 15 burpees

► 10 push-ups

► 10 squats

► 10 burpees

► 5 push-ups

► 5 squats

► 5 burpees

Total time ....

PUSH-UP

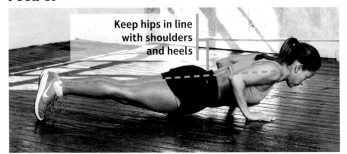

Keep hips in line with shoulders and heels

Start in a high plank position. Keep your hips in line with your heels and shoulders. Bend your elbows to lower your chest towards the floor until your elbows are bent to 90 degrees. Then straighten your arms. That is one rep.

SQUAT

Stand with your feet hip-width apart. Push your hips back until your thighs are parallel to the floor. Then push through your heels and extend your legs to return to standing. That is one rep.

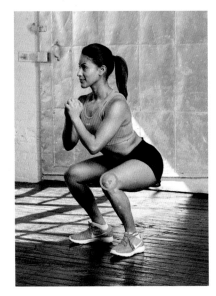

BURPEE

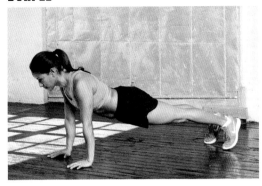

1 Place your feet hip-width apart, crouch down, and place your hands on the floor in front of your toes. Jump your feet back to a high plank position, then immediately jump forwards to the crouched position.

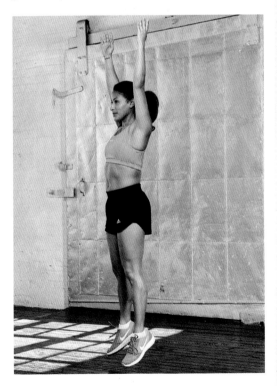

2 Quickly jump off the floor and reach your hands towards the ceiling. That is one rep.

IDENTIFY YOUR PROGRAMME

After completing the timed assessment on the opposite page, identify the programme that matches your results. Start your training at that level.

Total time
**OVER
6 MINS**

LEVEL 1

For those new to the gym or out of practice

▶ Build a foundation for more advanced strength training

▶ Focus on proper movement patterns

▶ Begin with your bodyweight or a low resistance on exercises until you are accustomed to the movement patterns

▶ Start working with a barbell during the last programme phase

Total time
4–6 MINS

LEVEL 2

For those who already have baseline fitness abilities

▶ Build on Level 1 movement patterns

▶ Challenge yourself with weights heavier than you've used before

▶ Begin working with a barbell straight away

Total time
**UNDER
4 MINS**

LEVEL 3

For those who feel extremely confident in the gym and have experience using a barbell

▶ Improve your strong foundation of cardio endurance

▶ Follow the programme exactly to bring focused structure for efficient results

▶ Push yourself through the intense and fun workouts

FOLLOWING A PROGRAMME

Once you've assessed your fitness and determined your programme level, you can get started on your weekly workouts. All programme levels follow the same structure. Before you begin, familiarize yourself with the programme structure and with the language used in the programmes. Begin with Weeks 1–4 of your assessed level.

PROGRAMME STRUCTURE

Each programme is 12 weeks long and is broken up into three 4-week phases. Each phase consists of a 7-day workout plan that you'll repeat for a total of 4 weeks. Then you'll move on to the next phase.

WEEKS 1–4
Develop baseline fitness and skills for the rest of the programme

WEEKS 5–8
Exercises increase in number and intensity

WEEKS 9–12
More metabolic conditioning to ensure results and prepare you for harder training

GET STRONG GLOSSARY

Chipper A style of metabolic conditioning where the number of reps per exercise decreases with each round or set.

Circuit A sequence of three or more exercises performed back to back, with a brief rest before repeating the sequence.

Climb the ladder A style of metabolic conditioning where the number of reps per exercise increases with each round or set.

EMOM Short for "every minute on the minute". A style of metabolic conditioning where you perform the prescribed number of reps of an exercise or a set of exercises at the top of every minute, then rest for the remainder of the minute.

Finisher A short metabolic conditioning circuit at the end of a workout day. Designed to completely fatigue your body with bursts of cardio work.

HIIT Short for "high-intensity interval training". Alternates between short periods of high-intensity cardio exercise and short periods of rest. A form of metabolic conditioning.

Main lift The main strength exercise in your workout day. A functional compound movement that uses a barbell or other weight (deadlift, squat, row, or press).

Metabolic conditioning A method of training that involves a high rate of work with little rest. It conditions your muscles to efficiently use your body's energy, making you fitter.

Reps Short for repetitions. The number of times you consecutively perform an exercise without resting.

Round One sequence or cycle of the exercises in a circuit.

Set One sequence or cycle of the exercises in a superset.

Superset A sequence of two exercises performed back to back, with a brief rest before repeating the sequence.

Tabata A style of metabolic conditioning where you perform 20 seconds of an exercise at your maximum effort, then rest for 10 seconds. Repeated for 8 rounds, or a total of 4 minutes.

THE PROGRAMMES

Programmes are divided into three 4-week phases. Each phase opens with a weekly schedule that outlines your workouts for the week. The following pages contain detailed workout instructions.

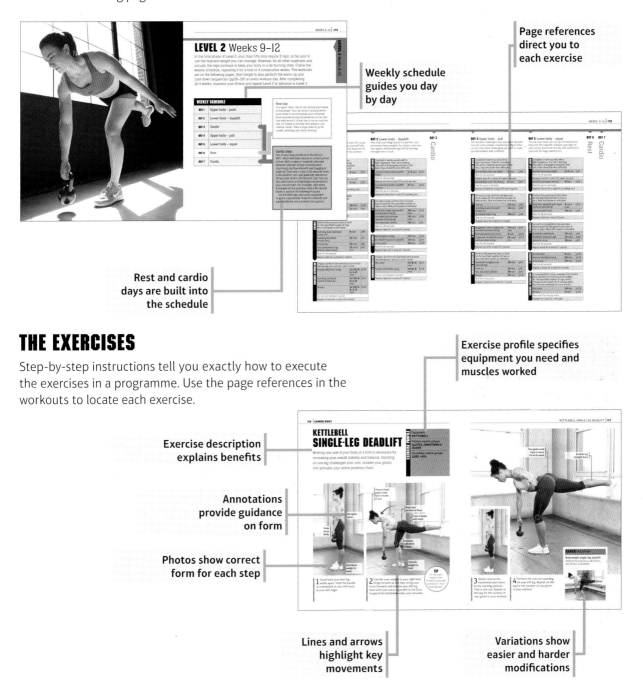

Page references direct you to each exercise

Weekly schedule guides you day by day

Rest and cardio days are built into the schedule

THE EXERCISES

Step-by-step instructions tell you exactly how to execute the exercises in a programme. Use the page references in the workouts to locate each exercise.

Exercise profile specifies equipment you need and muscles worked

Exercise description explains benefits

Annotations provide guidance on form

Photos show correct form for each step

Lines and arrows highlight key movements

Variations show easier and harder modifications

FOLLOWING A WORKOUT

Most workouts consist of a functional main lift (squat, deadlift, row, or press), followed by exercises that bring more definition to your muscles and incorporate cardio for metabolic conditioning. Before starting, read through the day carefully and make sure you know how to execute each exercise properly. Check that you have access to the equipment you need, and have a notebook handy to track your progress.

LEARN THE EXERCISES

Read through the workout and make sure you understand how the day is structured and exactly what to do for each part. If any exercise is unfamiliar, turn to the step-by-step exercise guide and learn how to perform it properly. Workouts are most effective and efficient if you can limit page-turning and reading in the midst of your exercise.

CHOOSE YOUR RESISTANCE

If you're new to using weights, it can be difficult to select your resistance. This is because each person has a unique amount of strength and endurance, and even two women of the same height and physique can differ greatly in the strength of their individual muscles. Finding the right weight for you will take some trial and error, and requires paying attention to cues from your body.

Before you begin a new exercise, look at the reps given for each set to assess roughly how heavy the weight should be. Lower reps (5–10) usually require heavier weights, and higher reps (12–20) usually require lighter weights.

Pick up a weight that feels manageable and begin your first set, being mindful of form and how challenging the weight feels. The last few reps of your set should be so challenging that you feel as though you cannot complete another rep. If you can easily perform 5–10 more reps with the same resistance, then it is too light. If you are struggling to complete the last 5 reps and your form begins to deteriorate, or you simply can't finish the set, then it is too heavy. Adjust the weight as needed until you find a resistance that feels right.

Over the course of the programme, you may notice the specified number of reps for a particular exercise decreasing – this is your cue to use heavier weights. If you notice the specified number of reps increasing, you still need to increase the weight a little bit to challenge your muscular endurance. The goal is to get stronger by gradually selecting heavier weights.

TIPS FOR SELECTING RESISTANCE

▶ **Begin with a light load.** Use lighter weights if you are new to the exercise or if you haven't done it recently.

▶ **Focus on form.** You should be able to maintain good form for every rep, even if it is challenging.

▶ **Pay attention to the final reps.** To make progress, the final reps of a set, especially the last set, should feel very difficult – almost as if you can't do any more.

▶ **Increase weight when you don't struggle.** If you can complete all sets and reps without struggling, increase the weight the next time you do the exercise.

▶ **Compete with yourself, not others.** Strive to improve your own strength, and don't worry about what other people are lifting.

TRACK YOUR PROGRESS

Keeping a record of your workouts holds you accountable to your programme and helps you see tangible evidence of your growing strength. Keep a notebook to write down your workouts, the resistance you used for each exercise, and details about how your workout generally felt. You can also measure your progress by taking week-by-week photographs, noticing the fit of your clothes, or taking body measurements (waist, hips, etc).

LEVEL 2

WEEKS 5–8: DAY 5 (4 January)

MAIN LIFT			
Barbell front squat	**Weight used**	**Reps**	**Notes**
Set 1 (warm-up)	30kg	**5**	
Set 2 (warm-up)	30kg	**5**	
Set 3 (working)	35kg	**8**	Slightly too heavy; was losing good form by the last set – try 32.5kg next week.
Set 4 (working)	35kg	**7**	
Set 5 (working)	35kg	**6**	

CIRCUIT			
3 rounds	**Weight used**	**Reps**	**Notes**
Single-leg kettlebell deadlift	1 kettlebell 10kg	**10/leg**	
Dumbbell sumo squat	1 dumbbell 20kg	**12**	Final reps didn't feel as challenging – increase weight to 22.5kg next week.
Jump squat	Bodyweight	**10**	

WARM UP

A good warm-up before your training session activates your muscles and prepares them for better, injury-free performance. Perform these dynamic stretches and metabolic movements before you start every workout to wake up your central nervous system and increase blood flow and oxygen to your muscles.

THE ROUTINE

This dynamic exercise sequence primes your muscles for effective training. Perform these exercises back to back for the specified number of reps or seconds before starting your workout.

WARM-UP		
Walkout	**8** reps	
Plank hip opener and T-spine rotation (alternating)	**10** reps	
Lateral hip opener (alternating)	**16** reps	
Reverse lunge with reach (alternating)	**16** reps	
Jumping jack	**30** secs	

WALKOUT

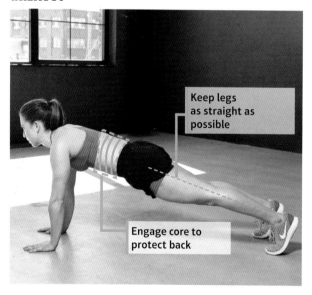

Keep legs as straight as possible

Engage core to protect back

Stand with your feet hip-width apart. With your legs straight, hinge at the hips, and place your hands on the floor in front of your toes. Walk your hands forwards until you are in a high plank position, letting your heels come off the floor. Then walk your hands back to your toes. That is one rep.

PLANK HIP OPENER AND T-SPINE ROTATION

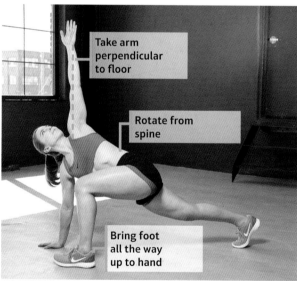

Take arm perpendicular to floor

Rotate from spine

Bring foot all the way up to hand

Begin in a high plank position. Bring your left foot up to the outside of your left hand. Lift your left arm, rotate your spine to the left, and extend your left arm to the ceiling, opening up your chest. Pause for a second, then return to the high plank position. That is one rep. Repeat on the other side.

LATERAL HIP OPENER

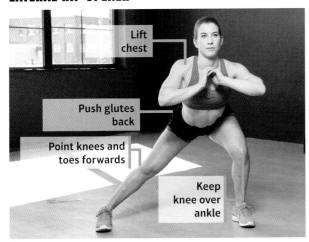

Lift chest

Push glutes back

Point knees and toes forwards

Keep knee over ankle

Stand with your feet wide, toes facing forwards. Keep your right leg straight, bend your left leg, and push your hips back. Feel a stretch in your right hip and leg. Then return to the starting position. That is one rep. Repeat on the other side.

REVERSE LUNGE WITH REACH

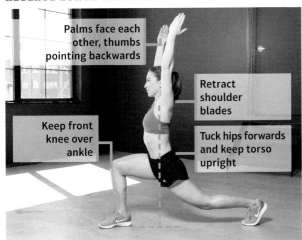

Palms face each other, thumbs pointing backwards

Retract shoulder blades

Keep front knee over ankle

Tuck hips forwards and keep torso upright

Stand with your feet hip-width apart. Step your left leg far back, and bend both knees until your right thigh is parallel to the floor. Reach your arms overhead. Hold the position firmly for a moment, then return to the starting position. That is one rep. Repeat on the opposite side.

JUMPING JACK

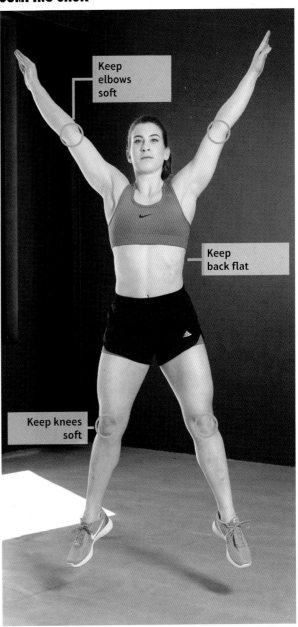

Keep elbows soft

Keep back flat

Keep knees soft

Stand with your feet together and rest your arms at your sides. In one motion, jump your feet out wider than shoulder-width apart, landing on the balls of your feet, and swing your arms out to the sides and overhead. Then immediately jump back to the starting position. That is one rep. Repeat quickly.

COOL DOWN

It is important to bring your body gradually back to a resting state after your training session. Perform this cool-down routine after every workout to lower your heart rate and prevent blood from pooling in your muscles. Proper cool-down stretches begin the muscle recovery process.

THE ROUTINE

This stretching sequence helps your body return to normal after training. Right after you finish any workout, perform the exercises back to back for the specified number of reps or seconds.

COOL DOWN		
Quad rocker	**10** reps	
Hip flexors stretch	**30** secs/leg	
Seated forward fold	**45** secs	
Supine spinal twist	**30** secs/side	
Chest stretch	**45** secs	

QUAD ROCKER

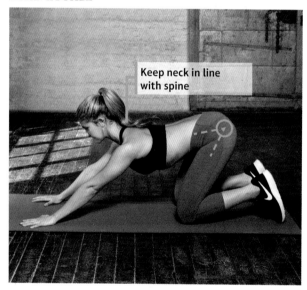

Keep neck in line with spine

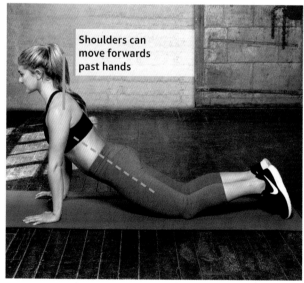

Shoulders can move forwards past hands

1 Begin in a tabletop position with your shoulders over your hands and your hips over your knees. Keep your hands planted, and push your hips back towards your heels. Briefly hold the stretch. Feel it in your shoulders, glutes, and lower back.

2 Keep your hands planted, and pull your body forwards to straighten your hips. Briefly hold the stretch. Feel it in your quads and hip flexors. That is one rep.

HIP FLEXORS STRETCH

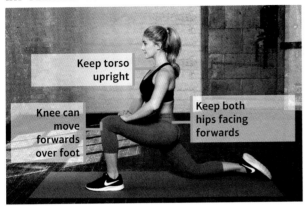

Keep torso upright

Knee can move forwards over foot

Keep both hips facing forwards

Begin in a half-kneeling position with your left leg forward and your right knee on the floor. Place your hands on your left thigh and lean forwards. Breathe steadily and hold the stretch. Feel it in your right hip flexors and quads. Repeat on the other side.

SEATED FORWARD FOLD

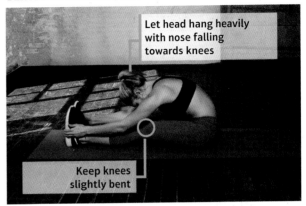

Let head hang heavily with nose falling towards knees

Keep knees slightly bent

Sit on the floor, extend your legs, and flex your feet. Reach forwards to grab the sides of your feet or calves. Breathe steadily and hold the stretch. Feel it in your hamstrings and spine.

SUPINE SPINAL TWIST

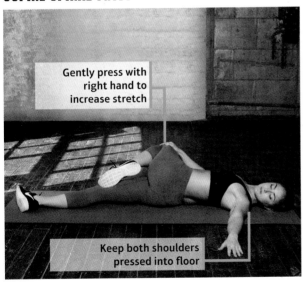

Gently press with right hand to increase stretch

Keep both shoulders pressed into floor

Lie on your back with your legs extended on the floor. Extend your left arm to the side and turn your head towards your left shoulder. Bend your left knee and use your right hand to pull it across your body to the right. Hold the stretch. Feel it in your lower back and glutes. Repeat on the other side.

CHEST STRETCH

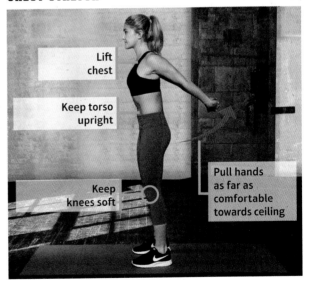

Lift chest

Keep torso upright

Keep knees soft

Pull hands as far as comfortable towards ceiling

Stand with your feet shoulder-width apart and bend your knees slightly. Clasp your hands together behind your back, palms facing out. Pull your arms back and up. Breathe steadily and hold the stretch. Feel it in your chest muscles.

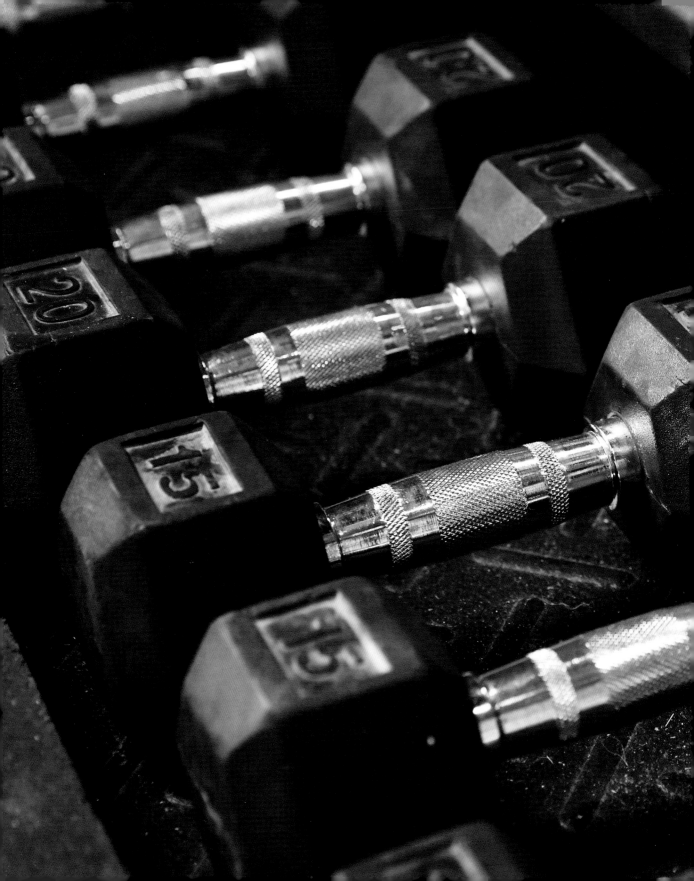

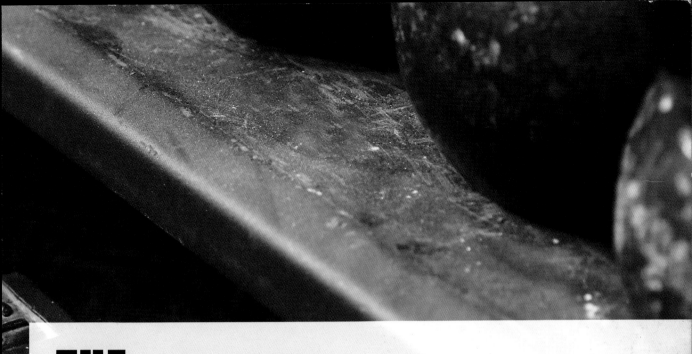

THE
EXERCISES

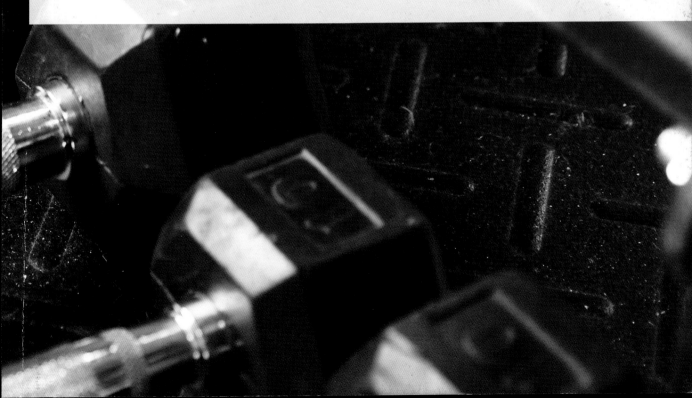

BICYCLE CRUNCH

This classic core-building exercise mimics the motion of riding a bicycle to target the front abdominals and oblique muscles, as well as your thighs. Perform the exercise slowly, concentrating on using your core for maximum toning effect.

EXERCISE PROFILE

Equipment
NONE

Primary muscle group
ABDOMINALS

Secondary muscle groups
GLUTES, QUADS, HAMSTRINGS

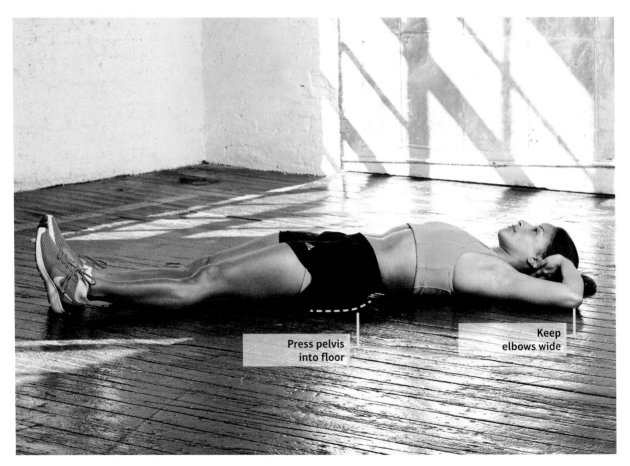

Press pelvis into floor

Keep elbows wide

1 Lie on the floor with your legs extended. Place your hands behind your head and point your elbows out to the sides.

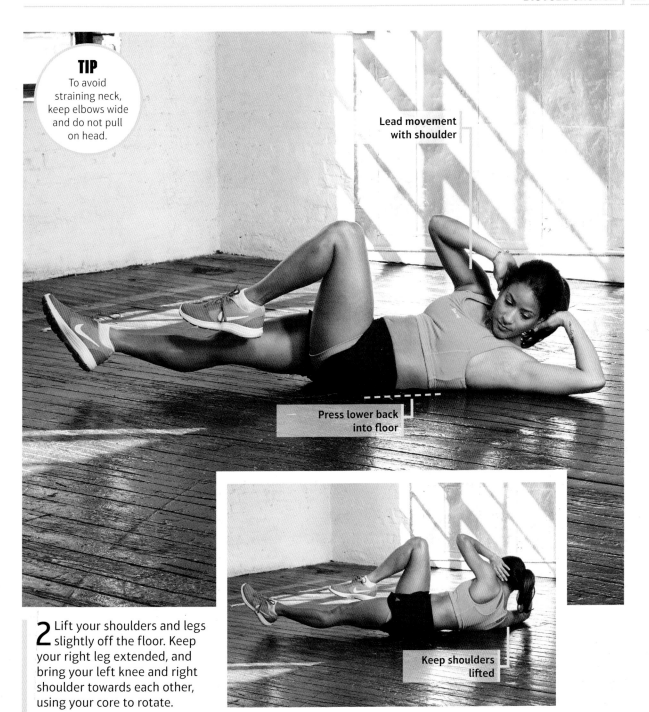

TIP
To avoid straining neck, keep elbows wide and do not pull on head.

Lead movement with shoulder

Press lower back into floor

Keep shoulders lifted

2 Lift your shoulders and legs slightly off the floor. Keep your right leg extended, and bring your left knee and right shoulder towards each other, using your core to rotate.

3 Rotate in the opposite direction, pulling your right knee and left shoulder towards each other while extending your left leg. That is one rep. Alternate crunching on each side for the number of reps given in your workout.

DUMBBELL TOE TOUCH

Isolate your upper abdominals with this floor-based core exercise. Extending your legs straight in the air creates a broad range of motion that adds intensity to a simple crunch and tones your core.

EXERCISE PROFILE

Equipment
DUMBBELL

Primary muscle group
ABDOMINALS

Secondary muscle groups
LOWER BACK, GLUTES, QUADS, HAMSTRINGS

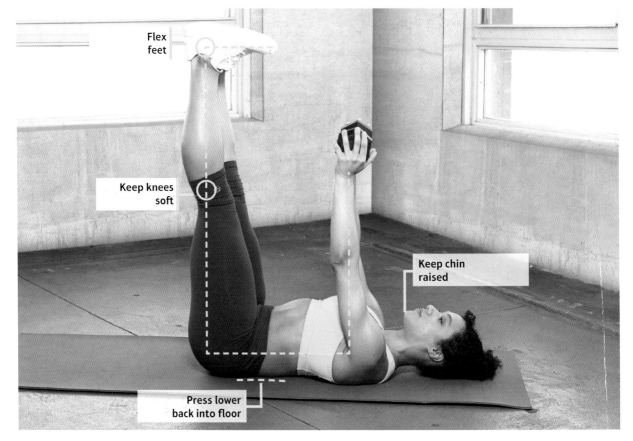

Flex feet

Keep knees soft

Keep chin raised

Press lower back into floor

1 Lie on your back and extend your legs straight up, with the soles of your feet facing the ceiling. Keep your legs and ankles pressed together, and bend your knees slightly. Hold the ends of one dumbbell with both hands and extend your arms straight up. Inhale.

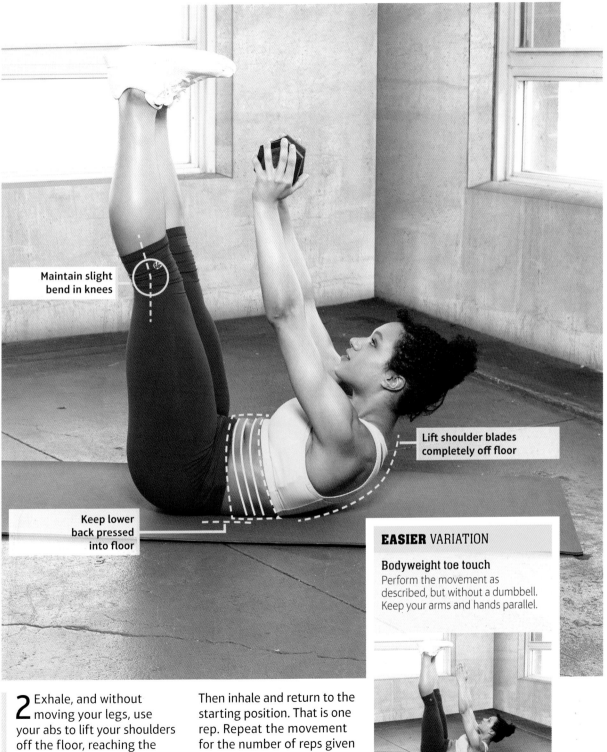

Maintain slight bend in knees

Lift shoulder blades completely off floor

Keep lower back pressed into floor

EASIER VARIATION

Bodyweight toe touch
Perform the movement as described, but without a dumbbell. Keep your arms and hands parallel.

2 Exhale, and without moving your legs, use your abs to lift your shoulders off the floor, reaching the dumbbell towards your toes.

Then inhale and return to the starting position. That is one rep. Repeat the movement for the number of reps given in your workout.

V-UP

This challenging movement targets the entire abdominal region and strengthens your lower back to protect the spine. The total-body reach also increases your flexibility and improves your balance. Try your best to touch your toes on every rep.

EXERCISE PROFILE

Equipment
NONE

Primary muscle group
ABDOMINALS

Secondary muscle groups
CORE, HIPS, QUADS

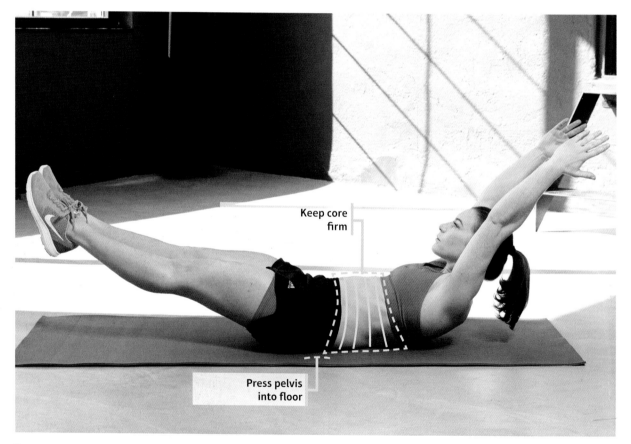

Keep core firm

Press pelvis into floor

1 Lie on your back, extend your legs, and lift them off the floor. Extend your arms straight above your head, and lift your shoulders fully off the floor. Engage your core, and inhale.

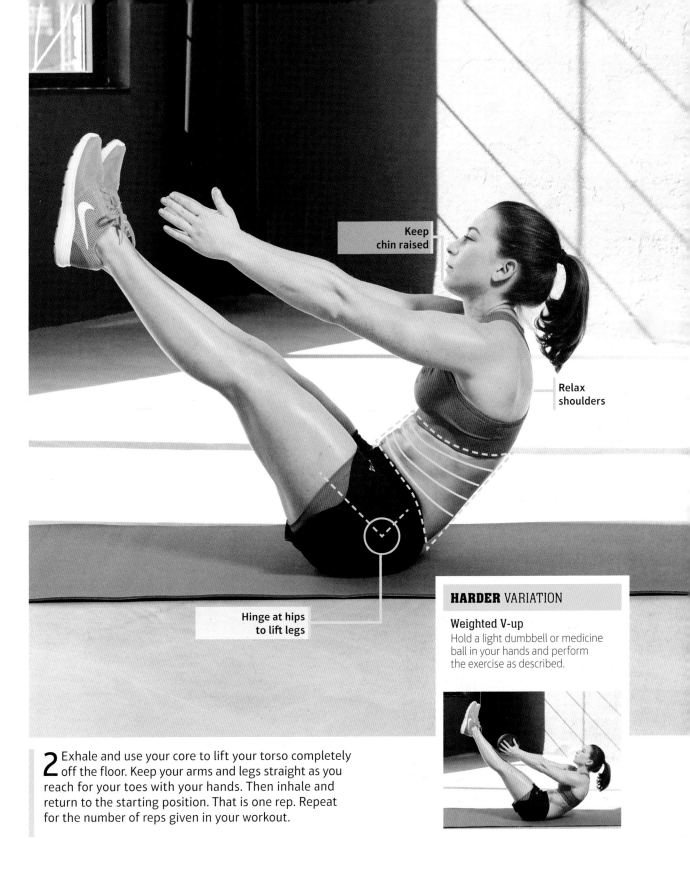

Keep
chin raised

Relax
shoulders

Hinge at hips
to lift legs

HARDER VARIATION

Weighted V-up
Hold a light dumbbell or medicine
ball in your hands and perform
the exercise as described.

2 Exhale and use your core to lift your torso completely
off the floor. Keep your arms and legs straight as you
reach for your toes with your hands. Then inhale and
return to the starting position. That is one rep. Repeat
for the number of reps given in your workout.

BUTTERFLY SIT-UP

A traditional sit-up can create tension in your hip flexors, but this variation of the sit-up opens up your hips and keeps them loose throughout your entire workout. Perform the movement slowly, letting the abdominal muscles do the work.

EXERCISE PROFILE

Equipment
NONE

Primary muscle group
ABDOMINALS

Secondary muscle groups
HIPS, GLUTES, UPPER BACK, SHOULDERS

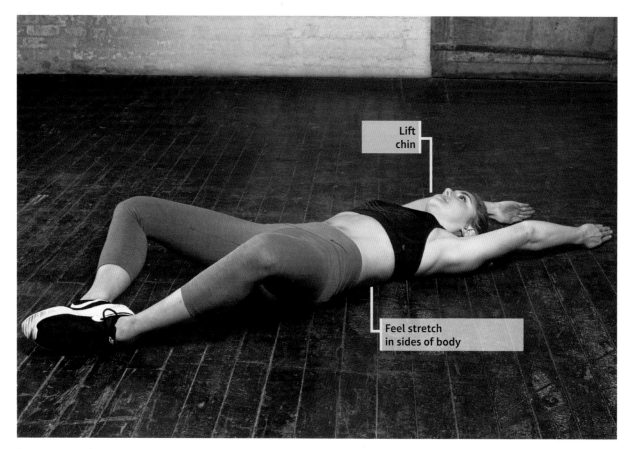

Lift chin

Feel stretch in sides of body

1 Lie on your back. Bend your knees, place the soles of your feet together, and pull your heels towards your body. Extend your arms above your head along the floor. Inhale.

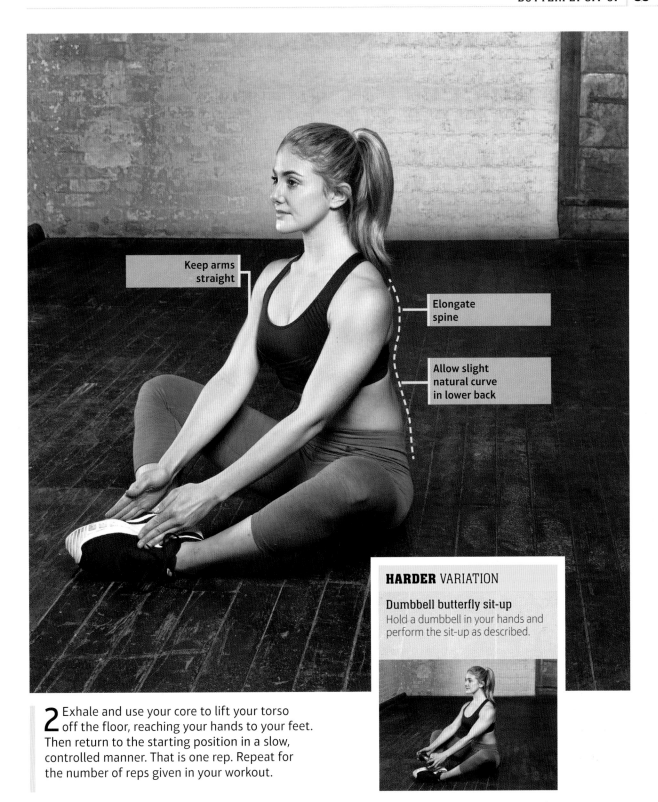

Keep arms straight

Elongate spine

Allow slight natural curve in lower back

HARDER VARIATION

Dumbbell butterfly sit-up
Hold a dumbbell in your hands and perform the sit-up as described.

2 Exhale and use your core to lift your torso off the floor, reaching your hands to your feet. Then return to the starting position in a slow, controlled manner. That is one rep. Repeat for the number of reps given in your workout.

SINGLE-ARM KETTLEBELL SIT-UP

By using one arm at a time for this weighted sit-up, you will increase strength and stability through your core. The movement strengthens your lower abdominals and obliques while stabilizing the shoulder muscles.

EXERCISE PROFILE

Equipment
KETTLEBELL

Primary muscle group
ABDOMINALS

Secondary muscle groups
SHOULDERS, TRICEPS

CAUTION

If you have lower back pain, bend your knees and place your feet on the floor.

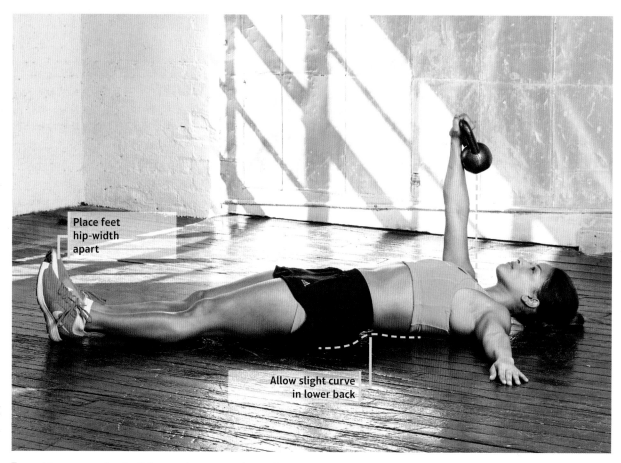

Place feet hip-width apart

Allow slight curve in lower back

1 Lie on your back with your legs straight. Hold a kettlebell in your right hand and extend your arm so the weight is above your shoulder, palm facing up. Keep your right arm in this position. Extend your left arm out to the side. Inhale.

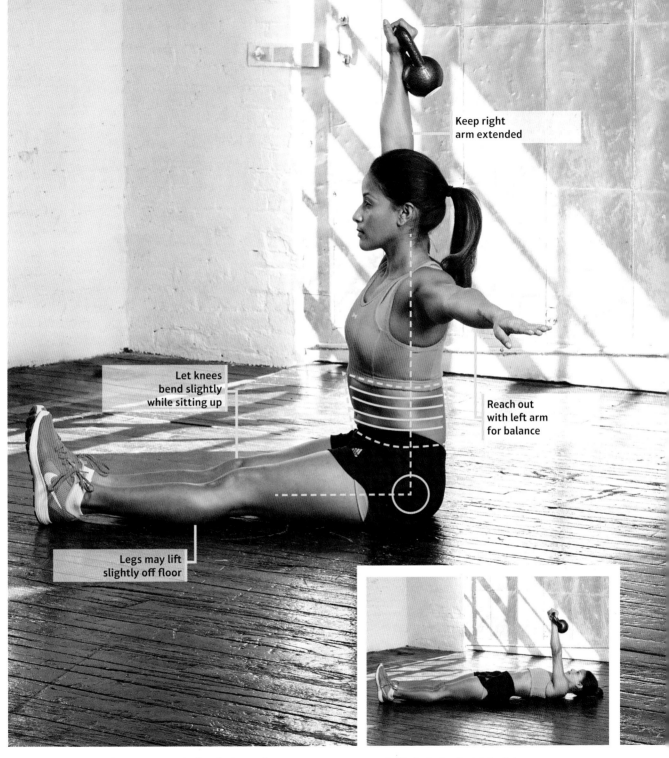

Keep right
arm extended

Let knees
bend slightly
while sitting up

Reach out
with left arm
for balance

Legs may lift
slightly off floor

2 Keep your right arm extended, exhale, and use your core to sit up until your torso is upright. Then slowly return to the starting position. That is one rep. Repeat with this arm for the number of reps given in your workout.

3 Switch the kettlebell to your left arm. Repeat the sit-up with this arm for the number of reps given in your workout.

KNEELING RING ROLLOUT

This advanced exercise is one of the best movements for strengthening your entire core. Using the rings will train your abdominal muscles to support your lower back and prevent your spine from hyperextending.

EXERCISE PROFILE

Equipment
RINGS

Primary muscle group
ABDOMINALS

Secondary muscle groups
SHOULDERS, GLUTES

CAUTION
Only go as far as you feel comfortable. Stop if you feel strain in your lower back.

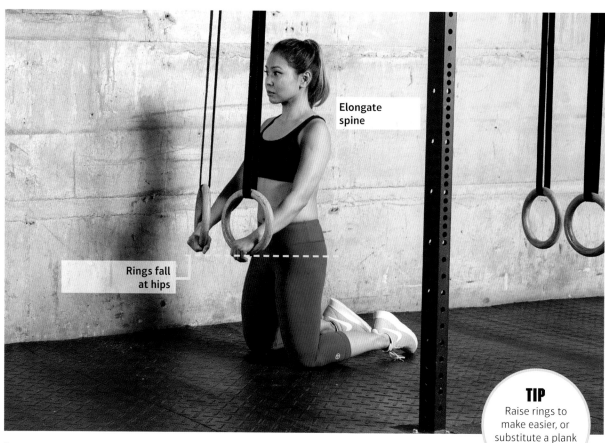

Elongate spine

Rings fall at hips

TIP
Raise rings to make easier, or substitute a plank to make harder.

1 Kneel behind the rings so they fall in front of your upper hips. Hold a ring in each hand, palms facing down, and relax your arms.

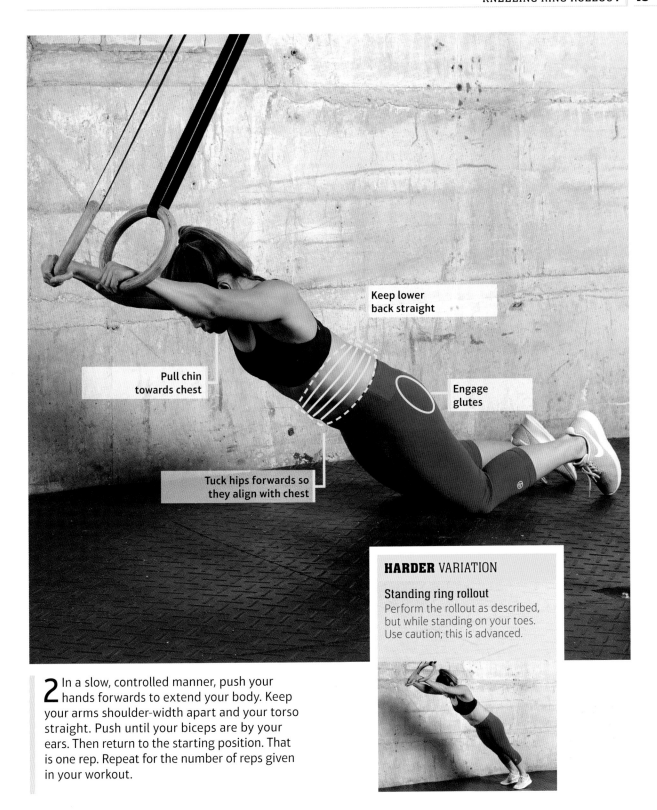

Keep lower back straight

Pull chin towards chest

Engage glutes

Tuck hips forwards so they align with chest

2 In a slow, controlled manner, push your hands forwards to extend your body. Keep your arms shoulder-width apart and your torso straight. Push until your biceps are by your ears. Then return to the starting position. That is one rep. Repeat for the number of reps given in your workout.

HARDER VARIATION

Standing ring rollout
Perform the rollout as described, but while standing on your toes. Use caution; this is advanced.

FOREARM PLANK LEG MARCH

Combining the plank with lower-body movement will make your abs and glutes burn. The plank position strengthens the transverse abdominals, the deep muscles of your core that stabilize the spine.

Equipment
NONE

Primary muscle groups
ABDOMINALS, GLUTES

Secondary muscle groups
SHOULDERS, UPPER LEGS

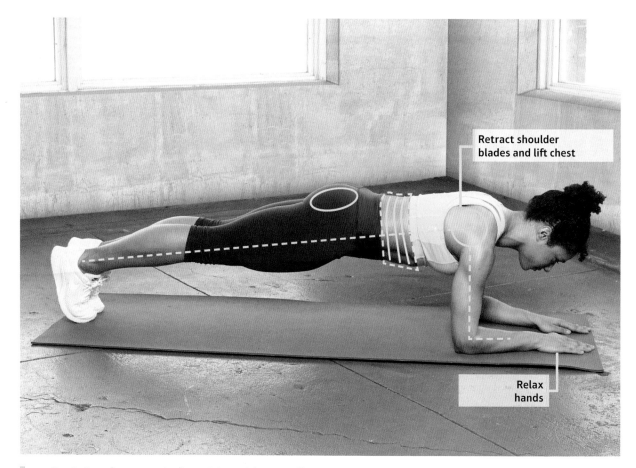

Retract shoulder blades and lift chest

Relax hands

1 Begin in a forearm plank position with your elbows below your shoulders. Align your hips with your heels and shoulders, and engage your core and glutes. Distribute your weight between your toes and forearms.

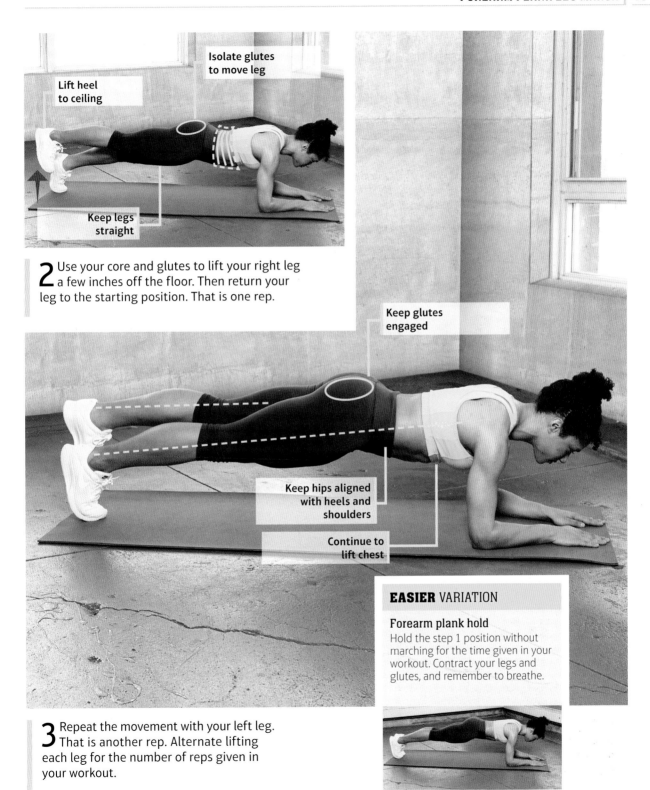

Isolate glutes
to move leg

Lift heel
to ceiling

Keep legs
straight

2 Use your core and glutes to lift your right leg a few inches off the floor. Then return your leg to the starting position. That is one rep.

Keep glutes
engaged

Keep hips aligned
with heels and
shoulders

Continue to
lift chest

EASIER VARIATION

Forearm plank hold
Hold the step 1 position without marching for the time given in your workout. Contract your legs and glutes, and remember to breathe.

3 Repeat the movement with your left leg. That is another rep. Alternate lifting each leg for the number of reps given in your workout.

HIGH PLANK SHOULDER TAP

Make a simple high plank more difficult by adding upper-body movement. Tapping one hand at a time to your opposite shoulder challenges your core to resist rotation and stabilize your position.

EXERCISE PROFILE

Equipment
NONE

Primary muscle groups
ABDOMINALS, SHOULDERS

Secondary muscle groups
TRICEPS, CHEST, LEGS

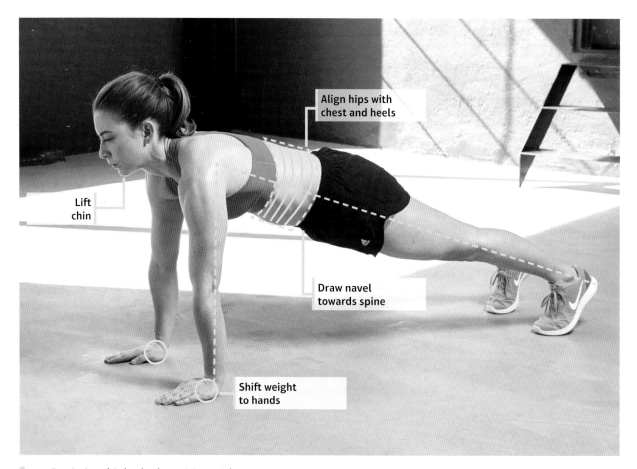

Align hips with chest and heels

Lift chin

Draw navel towards spine

Shift weight to hands

1 Begin in a high plank position with your shoulders above your hands and your toes hip-width apart. Shift your weight forwards into your hands and engage your core.

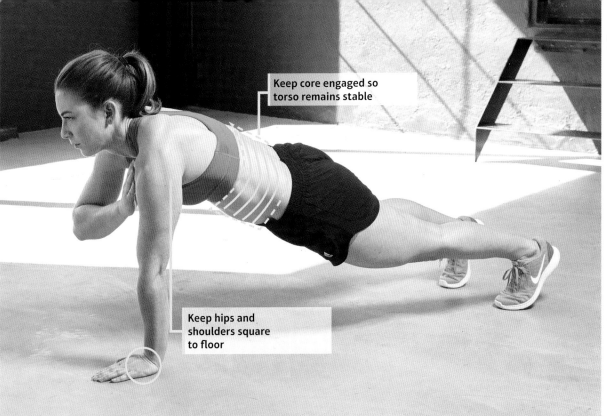

Keep core engaged so torso remains stable

Keep hips and shoulders square to floor

2 Without moving your torso, lift your right hand, shifting your weight to your left hand, and tap your left shoulder. Then return your right hand to the starting position. That is one rep.

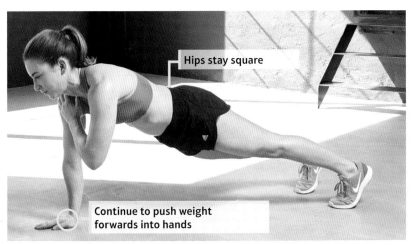

Hips stay square

Continue to push weight forwards into hands

3 Repeat the movement with your left hand. That is another rep. Tap alternately with each hand for the number of reps given in your workout.

EASIER VARIATION

High plank shoulder tap on knees
In step 1, place your knees on the floor. Perform the exercise as described, keeping a straight line from your head to knees.

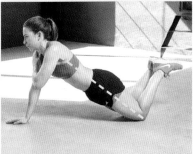

KETTLEBELL PLANK DRAG

With this variation of the high plank, you will challenge the stability of your core by dragging a weight back and forth under your body. This move will not only fire up your core, but also ignite your entire body.

EXERCISE PROFILE

Equipment
KETTLEBELL

Primary muscle group
ABDOMINALS

Secondary muscle groups
ARMS, SHOULDERS, CHEST

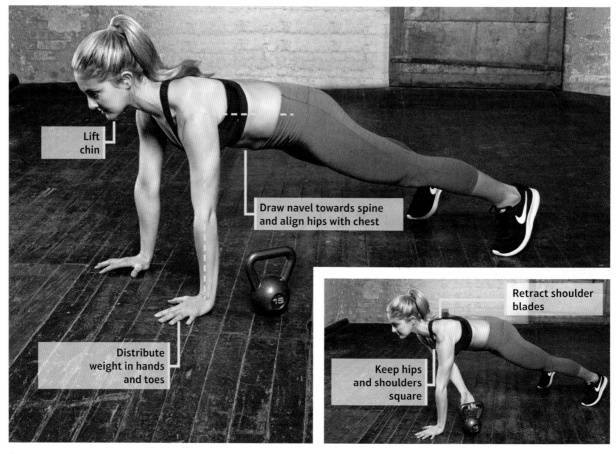

Lift chin

Draw navel towards spine and align hips with chest

Distribute weight in hands and toes

Retract shoulder blades

Keep hips and shoulders square

1 Begin in a high plank position with your shoulders above your hands and your toes wider than hip-width apart. Have a kettlebell placed just behind your left hand.

2 Without moving your torso, reach your right hand under your body and grab the handle of the kettlebell.

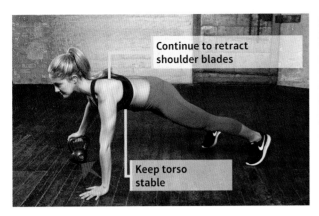

Continue to retract
shoulder blades

Keep torso
stable

3 Keep your hips and shoulders square, and pull the kettlebell along the floor to the right side of your body.

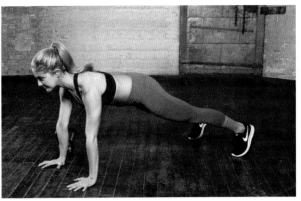

4 Return your right hand to the starting position, and redistribute your weight in your hands and toes. That is one rep.

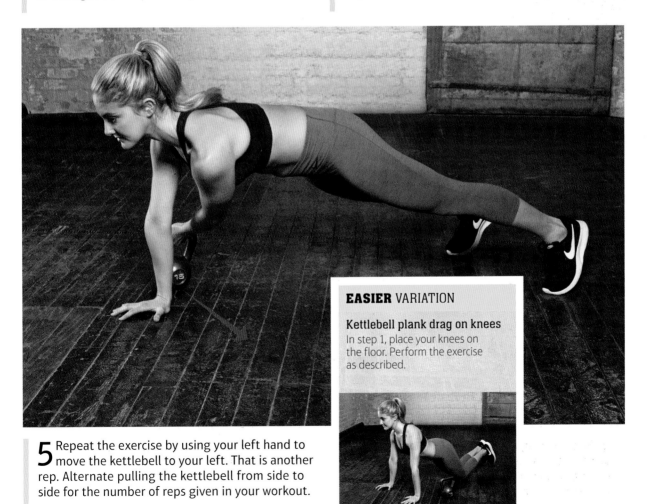

EASIER VARIATION

Kettlebell plank drag on knees
In step 1, place your knees on the floor. Perform the exercise as described.

5 Repeat the exercise by using your left hand to move the kettlebell to your left. That is another rep. Alternate pulling the kettlebell from side to side for the number of reps given in your workout.

SIDE PLANK
HIP DROP

This side plank improves the strength and stability of your core, which is the foundation of all efficient movement. The hip movement specifically targets your obliques, the abdominal muscles on the sides of your torso.

EXERCISE PROFILE

Equipment
NONE

Primary muscle group
OBLIQUES

Secondary muscle groups
SHOULDERS, GLUTES, HAMSTRINGS

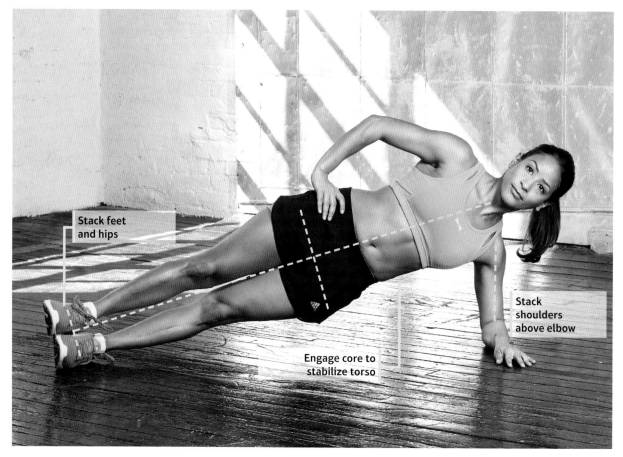

Stack feet and hips

Stack shoulders above elbow

Engage core to stabilize torso

1 Begin in a side plank position with your left forearm on the floor and left elbow bent to 90 degrees. Stack your right leg and hip directly over your left leg and hip. Lift your hips to form a straight line from your head to your heels. Place your right hand on your right hip.

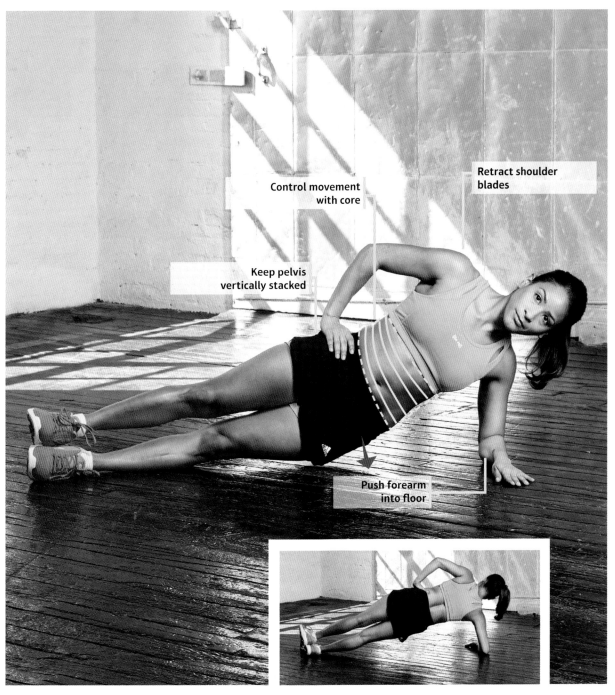

Retract shoulder blades

Control movement with core

Keep pelvis vertically stacked

Push forearm into floor

2 Use your core to lower your left hip to tap the floor. Then return to the starting position. That is one rep. Repeat on this side for the number of reps given in your workout.

3 Switch to the other side and perform the exercise by lowering your right hip to the floor. Repeat on this side for the number of reps given in your workout.

SIDE PLANK WARM HUG

This exercise adds a torso rotation to the side plank, forcing your core to work hard in order to stabilize your hips and maintain balance. The movement builds overall strength and stretches your chest muscles.

EXERCISE PROFILE

Equipment
NONE

Primary muscle group
OBLIQUES

Secondary muscle groups
CHEST, SHOULDERS, LEGS

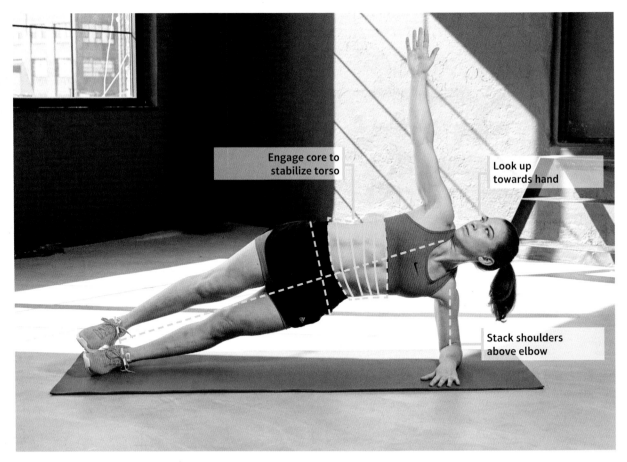

Engage core to stabilize torso

Look up towards hand

Stack shoulders above elbow

1 Begin in a side plank position with your left forearm on the floor and left elbow bent to 90 degrees. Stack your right leg and hip directly over your left leg and hip. Lift your hips to form a straight line from your head to your heels. Reach your right arm towards the ceiling.

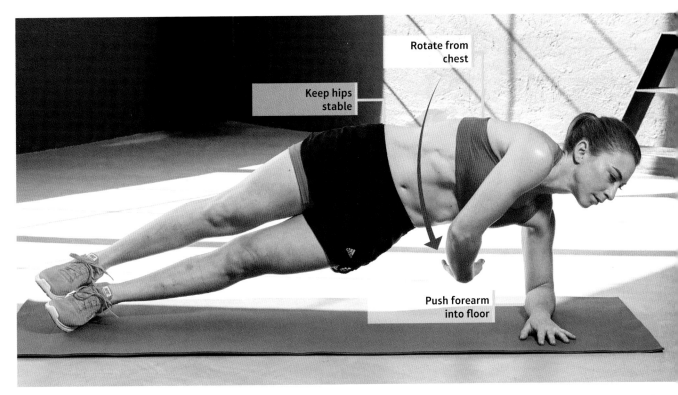

Rotate from chest

Keep hips stable

Push forearm into floor

2 Use your core to rotate your upper body and reach your right arm around your chest and past your hips, as if giving yourself a hug.

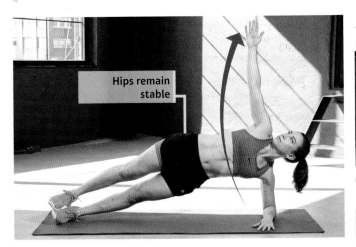

Hips remain stable

3 Return to the starting position. That is one rep. Repeat with your right arm for the number of reps given in your workout.

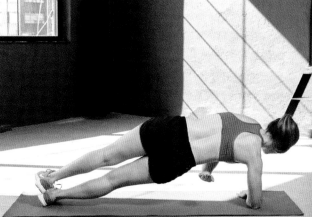

4 Switch to the opposite side and perform the exercise with your left arm. Repeat with this arm for the number of reps given in your workout.

MEDICINE BALL RUSSIAN TWIST

Adding a medicine ball to this core exercise increases resistance and quickly makes you stronger. The twisting movement targets your obliques, and the suspended leg position improves lower-body stabilization.

EXERCISE PROFILE

Equipment
MEDICINE BALL

Primary muscle group
ABDOMINALS

Secondary muscle groups
LOWER BACK, LEGS, SHOULDERS

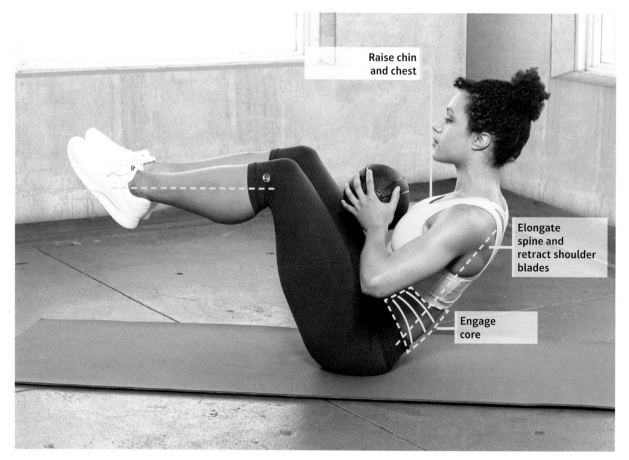

Raise chin and chest

Elongate spine and retract shoulder blades

Engage core

1 Sit on the floor and hold a medicine ball at your chest with both hands. Bend your knees and raise your feet until your shins are parallel to the floor. Lean back and engage your core to stay upright.

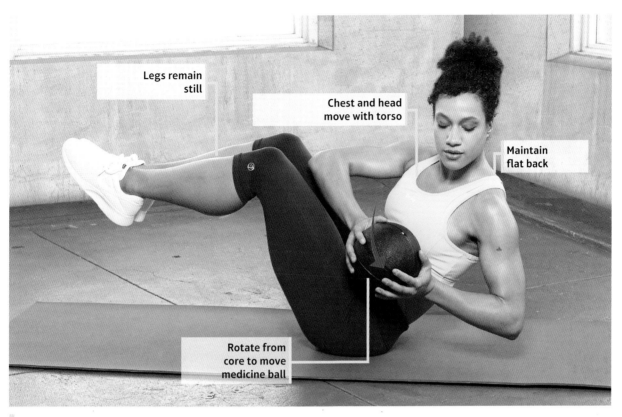

Legs remain still

Chest and head move with torso

Maintain flat back

Rotate from core to move medicine ball

2 Exhale and draw your navel towards your spine. Use your core to rotate your upper body, bringing the medicine ball to your left side.

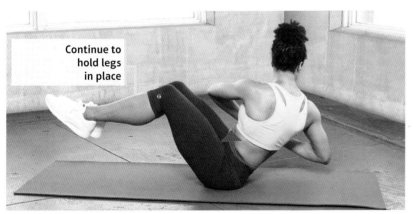

Continue to hold legs in place

3 Inhale and return to the centre, then exhale and rotate to your right. Inhale and return to the centre again. That is one rep. Alternate rotating to each side for the number of reps given in your workout, without letting your feet or back fall.

EASIER VARIATION

Bodyweight Russian twist
Perform the exercise as described, but without a medicine ball. Clasp your hands together. You can also rest your heels lightly on the floor.

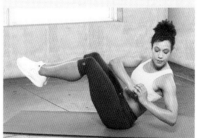

FAST MOUNTAIN CLIMBER

Boost your heart rate and metabolism while toning your core with this dynamic exercise. It primarily works the abs, which stabilize your shifting position. The faster you move, the more calories you will burn.

EXERCISE PROFILE

Equipment
NONE

Primary muscle group
ABDOMINALS

Secondary muscle groups
SHOULDERS, ARMS, LEGS, HIPS

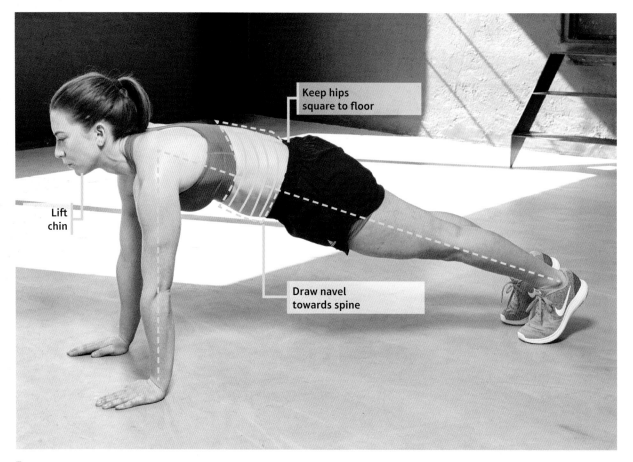

Keep hips square to floor

Lift chin

Draw navel towards spine

1 Begin in a high plank position with your shoulders above your hands and your toes hip-width apart. Distribute your weight evenly between your toes and hands.

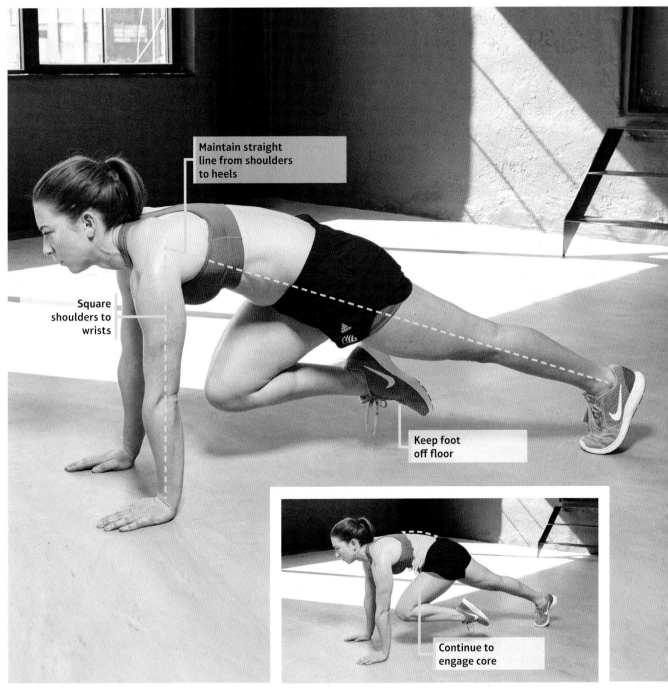

Maintain straight line from shoulders to heels

Square shoulders to wrists

Keep foot off floor

Continue to engage core

2 Quickly pull your right knee towards your chest while keeping your upper body stable and your shoulders above your wrists.

3 Quickly switch your legs, pulling your left knee to your chest and returning your right foot to the floor. Alternate raising each leg, maintaining a rapid pace for the time given in your workout.

SLOW CROSS MOUNTAIN CLIMBER

This movement intensifies the traditional mountain climber by adding a core rotation to isolate the obliques. Perform the exercise in a slow, controlled manner to sculpt your core and fire up your entire body.

EXERCISE PROFILE

Equipment
NONE

Primary muscle group
OBLIQUES

Secondary muscle groups
SHOULDERS, ARMS, HIPS, GLUTES, UPPER LEGS

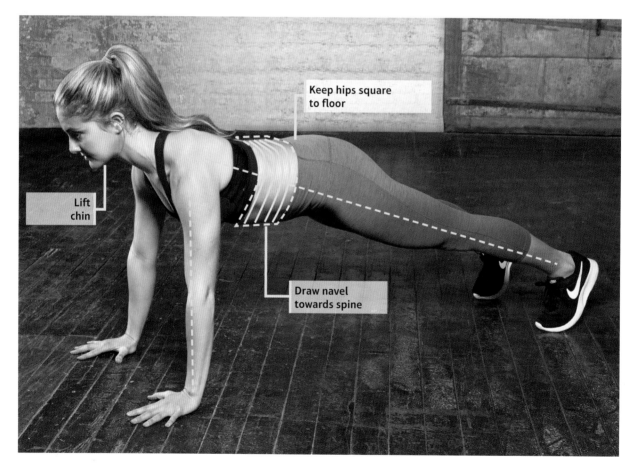

Keep hips square to floor

Lift chin

Draw navel towards spine

1 Begin in a high plank position with your shoulders above your hands and your toes hip-width apart. Distribute your weight evenly between your toes and hands. Inhale.

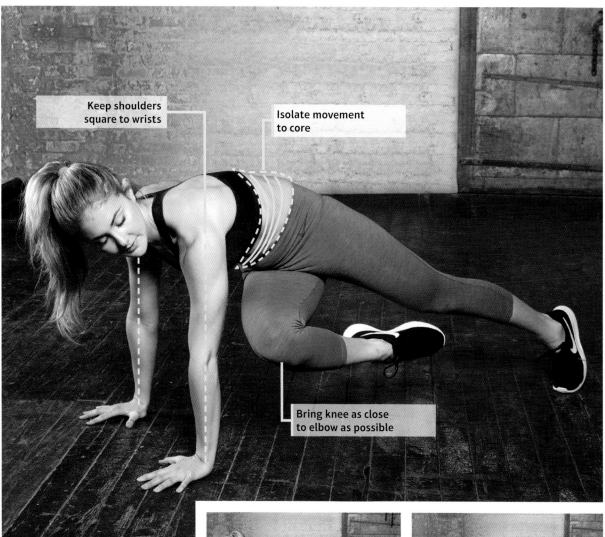

Keep shoulders
square to wrists

Isolate movement
to core

Bring knee as close
to elbow as possible

2 Exhale, and use your core to pull your right knee across your body, towards your left elbow. Maintain a stable upper body and keep your shoulders above your wrists.

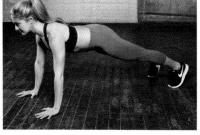

3 Inhale and return your right foot to the starting position. That is one rep.

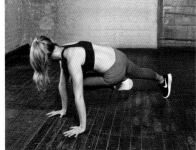

4 Exhale and repeat with your left leg. That is another rep. Alternate rotating to each side for the number of reps given in your workout.

KETTLEBELL FARMER'S WALK

Starting with a deadlift to pick up the kettlebells, then walking with the heavy weights, this exercise is one of the most functional for building total-body strength. Your forearms control the grip, and your core and shoulders work to hold your body upright under the resistance.

EXERCISE PROFILE

Equipment
KETTLEBELLS

Primary muscle groups
CORE, FOREARMS, SHOULDERS

Secondary muscle groups
LEGS, BACK

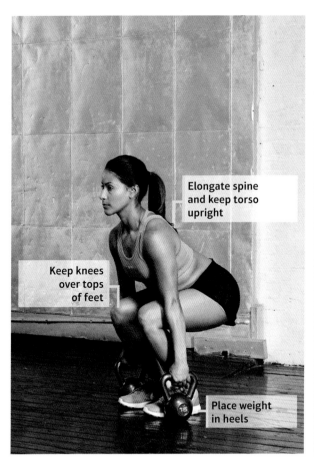

Keep knees over tops of feet

Elongate spine and keep torso upright

Place weight in heels

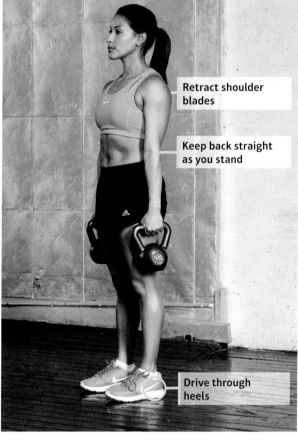

Retract shoulder blades

Keep back straight as you stand

Drive through heels

1 Stand between two kettlebells, positioned at the outside of each foot. Bend your knees, push your hips back, and grasp one kettlebell handle with each hand.

2 Push through your heels and stand up to lift the kettlebells off the floor. Hold them firmly at the sides of your body.

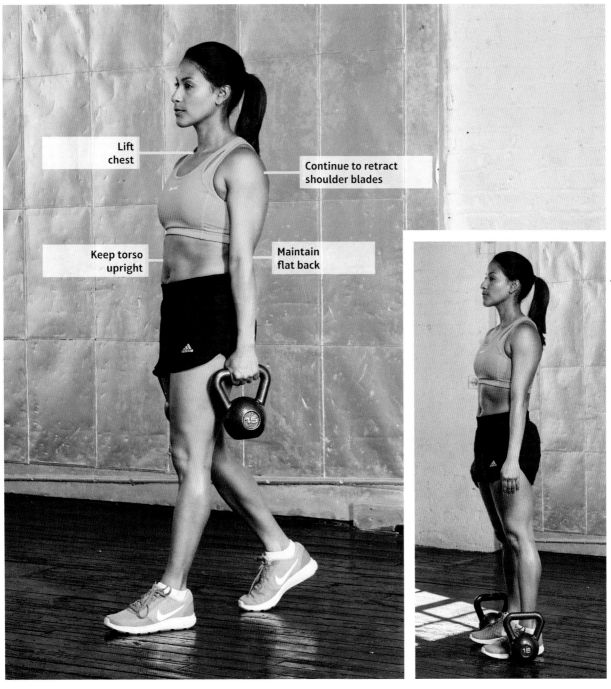

Lift chest

Continue to retract shoulder blades

Keep torso upright

Maintain flat back

3 Walk forwards with short, quick steps. Remember to breathe steadily as you move. Continue walking for the number of steps given in your workout.

4 Bend your knees and push your hips back, keeping your back flat. Set the kettlebells on the floor and return to standing.

STAGGERED STANCE SINGLE-ARM ROW

This rowing exercise isolates your upper back muscles, and the split stance recruits your core to stabilize your body. The single-arm focus helps to correct muscle imbalances caused by frequent sitting or reaching.

EXERCISE PROFILE

Equipment
DUMBBELL

Primary muscle groups
BACK, SHOULDERS

Secondary muscle groups
BICEPS, TRICEPS, CORE

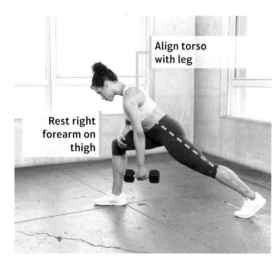

Align torso with leg

Rest right forearm on thigh

1 Stand with your feet shoulder-width apart and hold a dumbbell in your left hand. Step your left foot back into a staggered stance, and rise up onto the ball of your left foot. Hinge forwards at your hips and bend your right knee. Retract your shoulder blades.

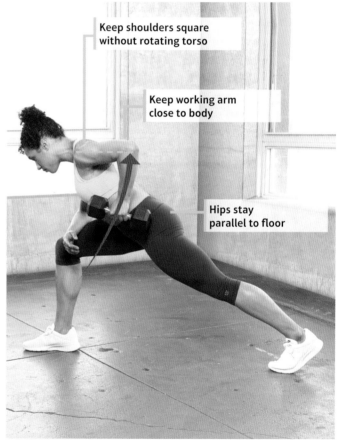

Keep shoulders square without rotating torso

Keep working arm close to body

Hips stay parallel to floor

2 Guided by your elbow, pull the dumbbell straight back and up, brushing your biceps along your torso, until the dumbbell is by your ribcage. Pause briefly at the top of the movement.

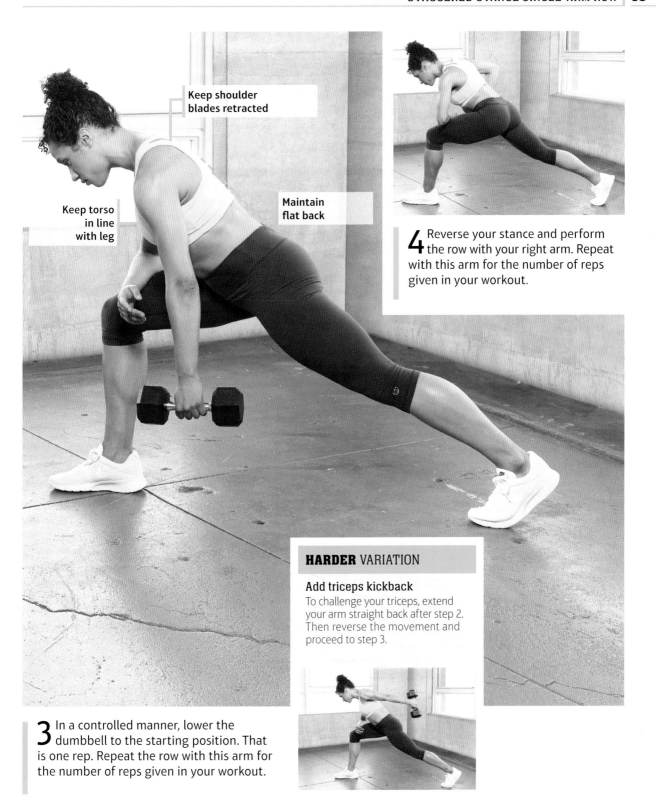

Keep shoulder blades retracted

Keep torso in line with leg

Maintain flat back

4 Reverse your stance and perform the row with your right arm. Repeat with this arm for the number of reps given in your workout.

HARDER VARIATION

Add triceps kickback
To challenge your triceps, extend your arm straight back after step 2. Then reverse the movement and proceed to step 3.

3 In a controlled manner, lower the dumbbell to the starting position. That is one rep. Repeat the row with this arm for the number of reps given in your workout.

DUMBBELL RENEGADE ROW

This advanced plank and row engages your entire body, with a particular focus on strengthening the back. It is a fantastic exercise for training your core to keep your hips, torso, and lower back in stable alignment.

EXERCISE PROFILE

Equipment
DUMBBELLS

Primary muscle groups
BACK, SHOULDERS, ABDOMINALS

Secondary muscle groups
BICEPS, TRICEPS

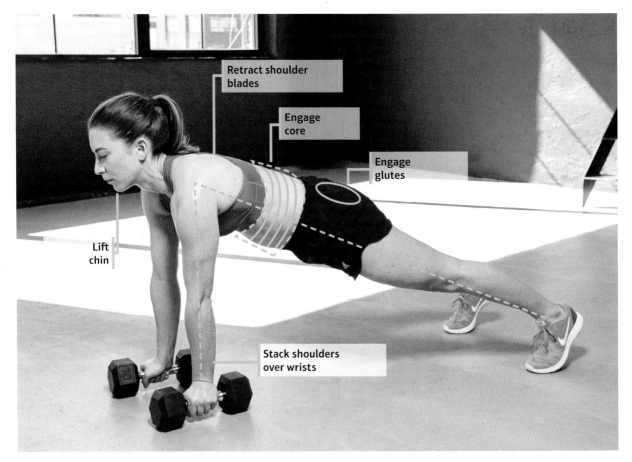

Retract shoulder blades

Engage core

Engage glutes

Lift chin

Stack shoulders over wrists

1 Hold a dumbbell in each hand and begin in a high plank position, with your shoulders above your hands and your toes wider than hip-width apart. Shift your weight to your toes. Inhale.

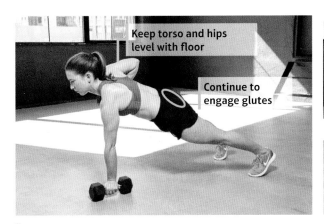

Keep torso and hips level with floor

Continue to engage glutes

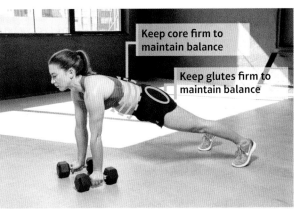

Keep core firm to maintain balance

Keep glutes firm to maintain balance

2 Exhale and pull the dumbbell in your right hand straight back and up, until it is by your ribcage. Pause briefly at the top of the movement.

3 Return the dumbbell to the starting position and redistribute your weight to your hands and toes. That is one rep.

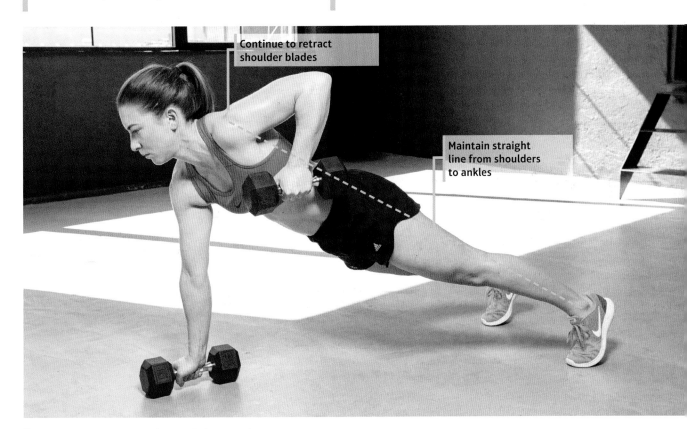

Continue to retract shoulder blades

Maintain straight line from shoulders to ankles

4 Repeat the row with your left arm. That is another rep. Alternate rowing with each arm for the number of reps given in your workout.

BARBELL BENT-OVER ROW

Your middle back is key for transferring power from the lower to upper body. This exercise begins with a deadlift, then you will move the bar up and down to strengthen your middle back. This also improves your fitness for other barbell movements, such as the bench press.

EXERCISE PROFILE

Equipment
BARBELL

Primary muscle groups
BACK, SHOULDERS

Secondary muscle groups
CORE, ARMS

CAUTION

Avoid this exercise if you have back issues. Do the Staggered stance single-arm row instead.

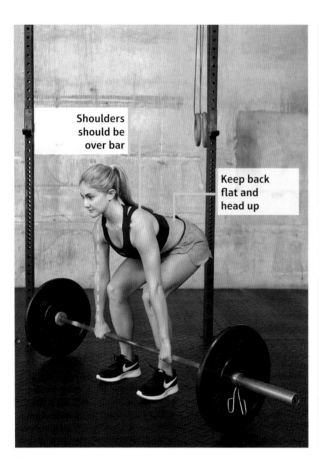

Shoulders should be over bar

Keep back flat and head up

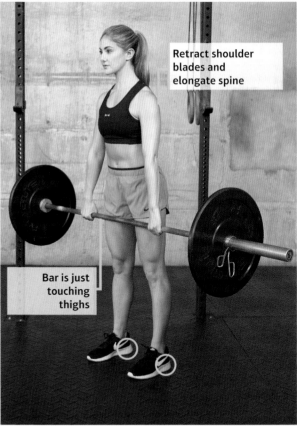

Retract shoulder blades and elongate spine

Bar is just touching thighs

1 Stand behind the barbell with your feet shoulder-width apart and the bar above your feet. Bend your knees and push your hips back. Grip the barbell with an overhand grip, slightly wider than shoulder width. Inhale.

2 Exhale and push through your heels to stand up, keeping your back straight, until your legs are extended and your torso is upright.

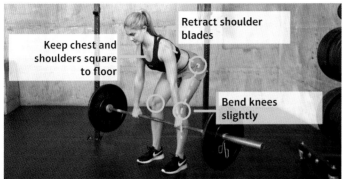

Keep chest and shoulders square to floor

Retract shoulder blades

Bend knees slightly

3 Hinge forwards at the hips, bring your chest forwards, and push your glutes back. Lower the barbell until it is below your knees. This is the starting position for the row.

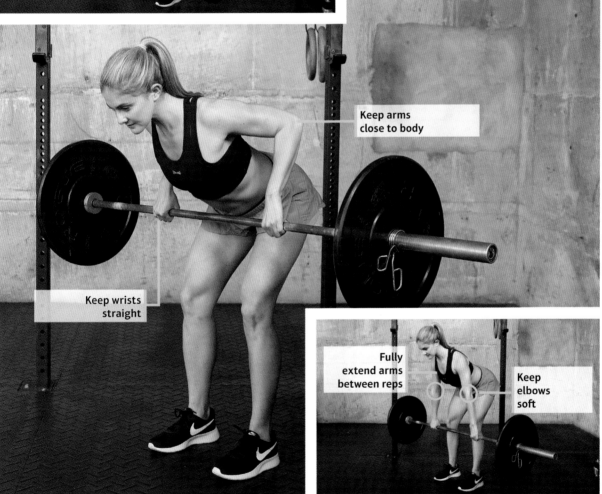

Keep arms close to body

Keep wrists straight

Fully extend arms between reps

Keep elbows soft

4 Exhale and use your mid-back to pull the bar up and back to your lower chest, guided by your elbows. Squeeze your shoulder blades at the top of the movement.

5 In a slow, controlled manner, lower your arms to the starting position. That is one rep. Repeat steps 4 and 5 for the number of reps given in your workout.

DUMBBELL UPRIGHT ROW

This foundational exercise sculpts your shoulders and will help you perform other upper-body exercises. Pulling the weights up while flaring out your elbows improves the mobility of your rotator cuff.

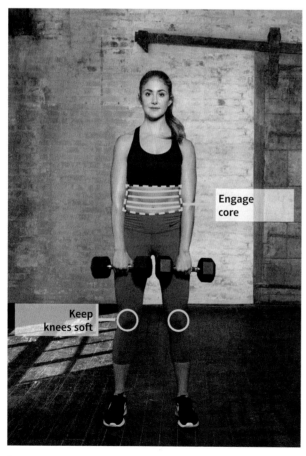

Engage core

Keep knees soft

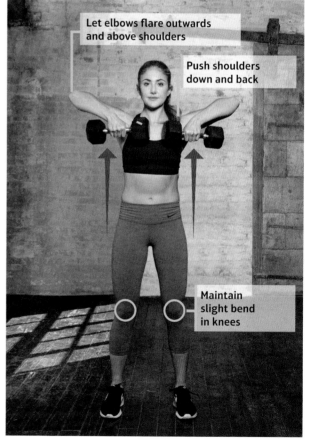

Let elbows flare outwards and above shoulders

Push shoulders down and back

Maintain slight bend in knees

1 Stand with your feet shoulder-width apart. With a dumbbell in each hand, hold your arms in front of you, palms facing your thighs. Bend your knees slightly and straighten your back.

2 In a slow, controlled manner, use your shoulders to pull the dumbbells up to your collarbone. Slowly return to the starting position. That is one rep. Repeat for the number of reps in your workout.

RING ROW

Using rings to row your body's weight prepares you for pull-ups. The total-body movement strengthens your upper back and arms. You can make this easier by walking your feet backwards, away from the rings, or make it more difficult by walking them forwards.

EXERCISE PROFILE

Equipment
RINGS

Primary muscle groups
UPPER BACK, BICEPS

Secondary muscle groups
SHOULDERS, TRICEPS, CORE

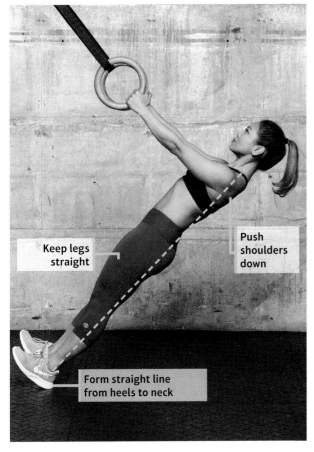

Keep legs straight

Push shoulders down

Form straight line from heels to neck

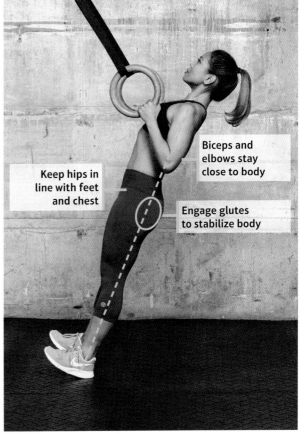

Keep hips in line with feet and chest

Biceps and elbows stay close to body

Engage glutes to stabilize body

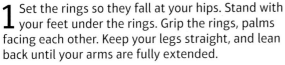

1 Set the rings so they fall at your hips. Stand with your feet under the rings. Grip the rings, palms facing each other. Keep your legs straight, and lean back until your arms are fully extended.

2 Draw your elbows straight back to pull your chest to the rings. Pause briefly, then return to the starting position. That is one rep. Repeat for the number of reps given in your workout.

BARBELL BENCH PRESS

The classic barbell bench press is crucial for building upper-body strength and defining your chest muscles. The movement helps prevent injury and corrects muscle imbalances between your chest and your back muscles.

EXERCISE PROFILE

Equipment
BENCH, BARBELL

Primary muscle group
CHEST

Secondary muscle groups
TRICEPS, BICEPS, SHOULDERS

CAUTION

Recruit a spotter if you are new to this exercise.

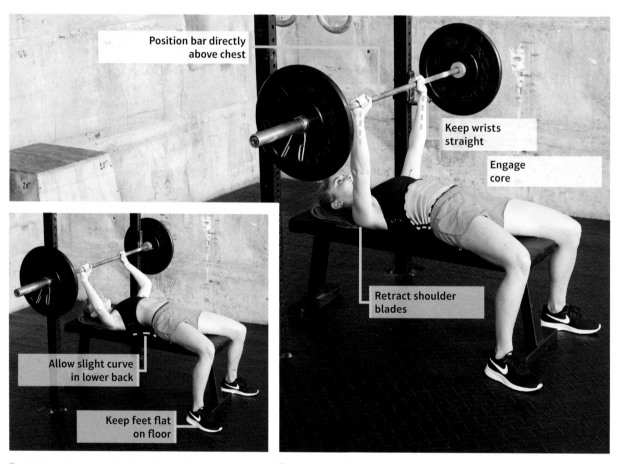

Position bar directly above chest

Keep wrists straight

Engage core

Retract shoulder blades

Allow slight curve in lower back

Keep feet flat on floor

1 Lie down on the bench with your shoulders beneath the bar. Hold the bar with your hands shoulder-width apart, palms facing away from you.

2 Straighten your arms to unrack the bar. Hover the bar above your chest. Do not let the bar drift forwards or backwards. Exhale.

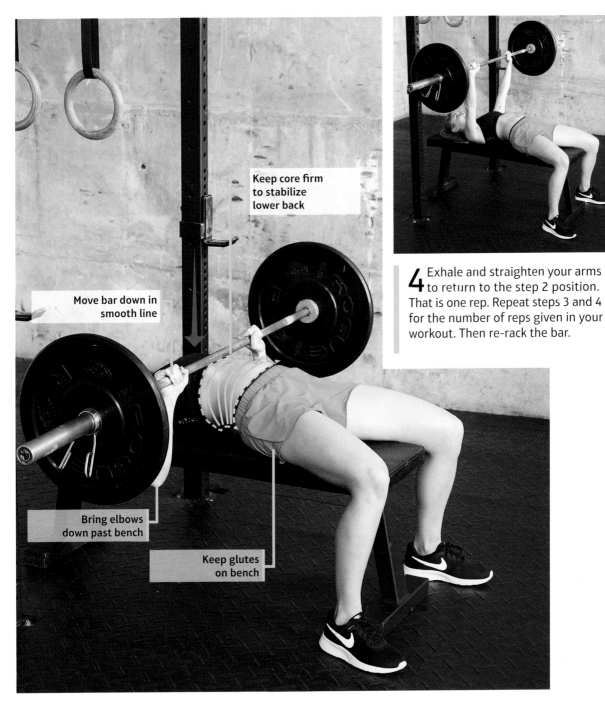

Keep core firm to stabilize lower back

Move bar down in smooth line

Bring elbows down past bench

Keep glutes on bench

4 Exhale and straighten your arms to return to the step 2 position. That is one rep. Repeat steps 3 and 4 for the number of reps given in your workout. Then re-rack the bar.

3 Inhale, and in a controlled manner, use your chest muscles to lower the bar and gently tap your lower chest. (Do not let the bar bounce off your body.)

SINGLE-ARM HALF-KNEELING KETTLEBELL PRESS

Tone your shoulders and develop your core with one exercise. The single-arm press targets your back and shoulder muscles, while the half-kneeling stance engages core muscles to stabilize and maintain balance.

EXERCISE PROFILE

Equipment
KETTLEBELL

Primary muscle groups
SHOULDERS, BACK

Secondary muscle groups
CORE, TRICEPS

CAUTION
To avoid straining your neck, look straight ahead and lift your chin.

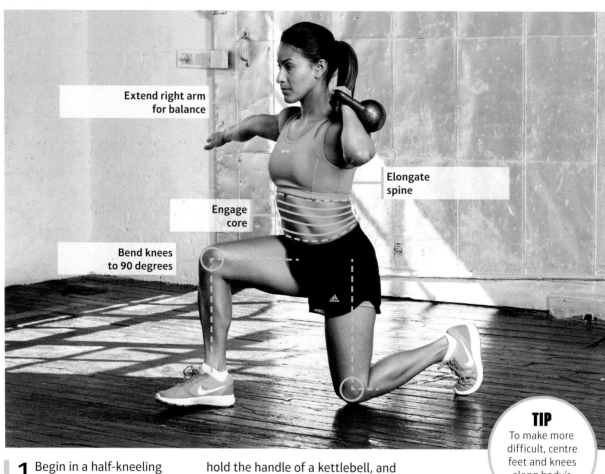

Extend right arm for balance

Elongate spine

Engage core

Bend knees to 90 degrees

1 Begin in a half-kneeling position with your right leg forward and your left knee on the ground. In your left hand, hold the handle of a kettlebell, and rest the weight on the back of your shoulder. Extend your right arm to the side or place it on your hip.

TIP
To make more difficult, centre feet and knees along body's midline.

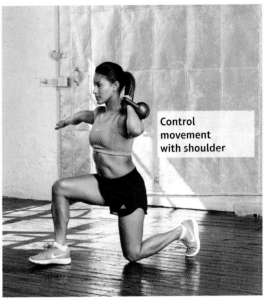

Control movement with shoulder

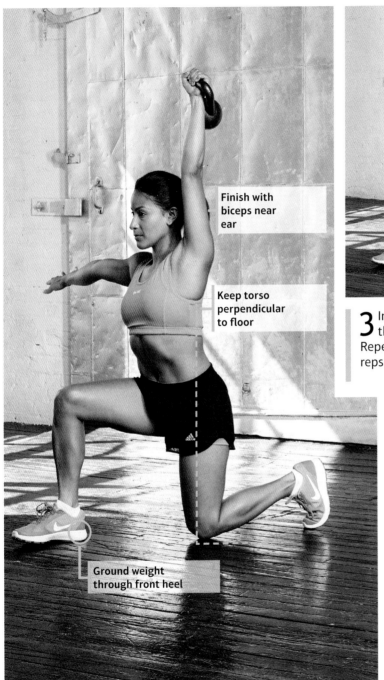

Finish with biceps near ear

Keep torso perpendicular to floor

Ground weight through front heel

3 In a controlled manner, return to the starting position. That is one rep. Repeat with this arm for the number of reps given in your workout.

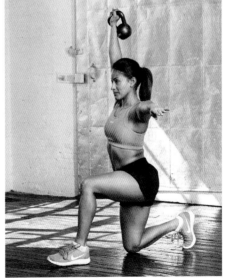

2 Exhale and use your shoulder to press the kettlebell straight up.

4 Reverse your stance and perform the exercise with your right arm. Repeat with this arm for the number of reps given in your workout.

STANDING DUMBBELL SHOULDER PRESS

This press builds strength in your shoulder muscles as you work to stabilize the independent weights. By performing the movement in a standing position, you engage your core muscles to maintain control and balance.

1 Stand with your feet shoulder-width apart. Hold a dumbbell in each hand at chin height, with your palms facing forwards. Inhale.

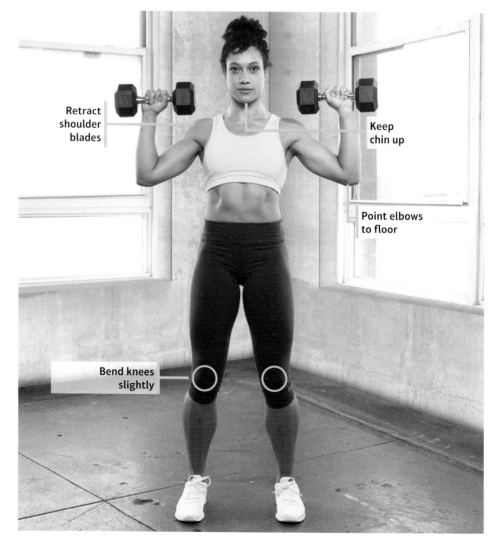

Retract shoulder blades

Keep chin up

Point elbows to floor

Bend knees slightly

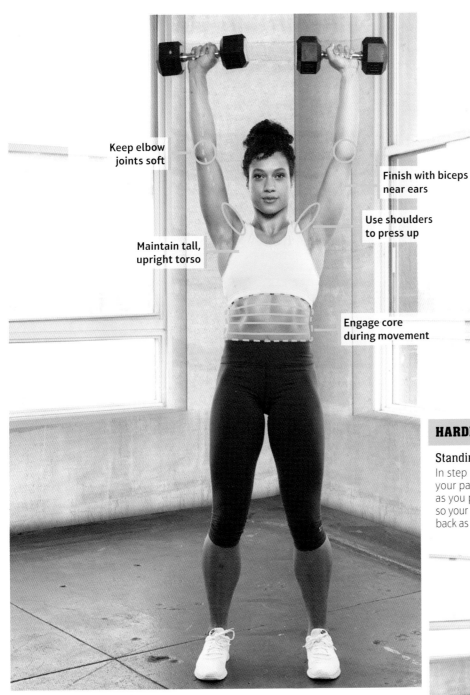

Keep elbow joints soft

Finish with biceps near ears

Use shoulders to press up

Maintain tall, upright torso

Engage core during movement

HARDER VARIATION

Standing dumbbell Arnold press

In step 1, hold the dumbbells with your palms towards you. In step 2, as you press up, rotate your hands so your palms face forwards. Rotate back as you lower them.

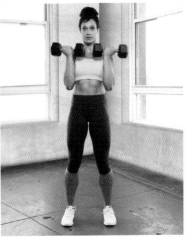

2 Exhale and use your shoulders to press the dumbbells straight up. Then, in a controlled manner, return to the starting position. That is one rep. Repeat for the number of reps given in your workout.

LYING DUMBBELL CHEST FLY

Lying on a bench allows for a full range of motion as you spread your arms wide, isolating and strengthening the chest muscles. This movement also keeps the rotator cuff flexible and stable, which helps prevent injury.

EXERCISE PROFILE

Equipment
DUMBBELLS, BENCH

Primary muscle group
CHEST

Secondary muscle groups
SHOULDERS, BACK, BICEPS

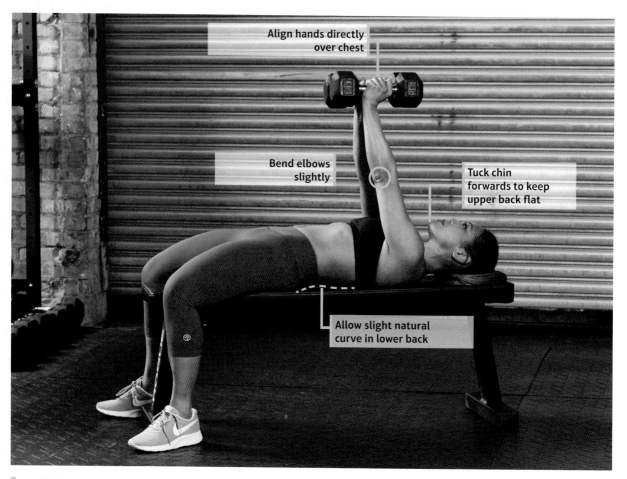

Align hands directly over chest

Bend elbows slightly

Tuck chin forwards to keep upper back flat

Allow slight natural curve in lower back

1 Lie on your back on a flat bench and hold a dumbbell in each hand. Fully extend your arms above your chest, palms facing each other.

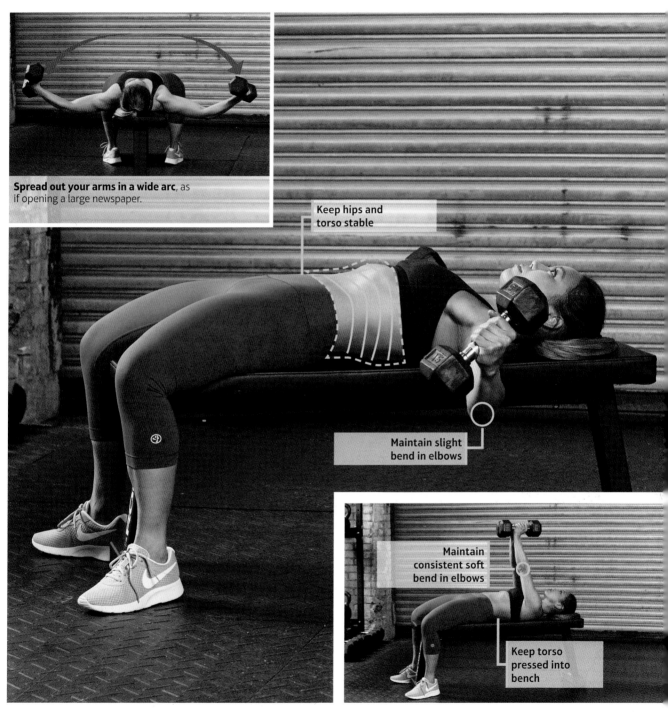

Spread out your arms in a wide arc, as if opening a large newspaper.

Keep hips and torso stable

Maintain slight bend in elbows

Maintain consistent soft bend in elbows

Keep torso pressed into bench

2 In a controlled manner, use your chest muscles to open up your arms and lower the dumbbells until your arms are nearly parallel to the floor.

3 Exhale and pull your arms back to the starting position. That is one rep. Repeat for the number of reps given in your workout.

BARBELL OVERHEAD PRESS

Also known as the military press, this advanced exercise is a great upper-body and core-building drill. The movement will increase your overall strength, defining your shoulders and improving torso and leg stability.

EXERCISE PROFILE

Equipment
BARBELL

Primary muscle groups
SHOULDERS, UPPER BACK

Secondary muscle groups
CORE, LEGS, TRICEPS

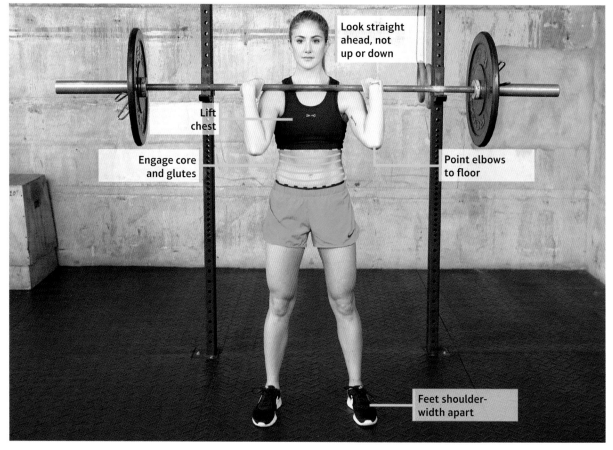

Look straight ahead, not up or down

Lift chest

Engage core and glutes

Point elbows to floor

Feet shoulder-width apart

1 Set the bar just below shoulder height on the rack. Grasp the bar with your hands slightly wider than shoulder-width apart, palms facing up. Straighten your knees and step forwards to unrack the bar. Place your feet shoulder-width apart. Rest the bar on your collarbone. Retract your shoulder blades. Inhale.

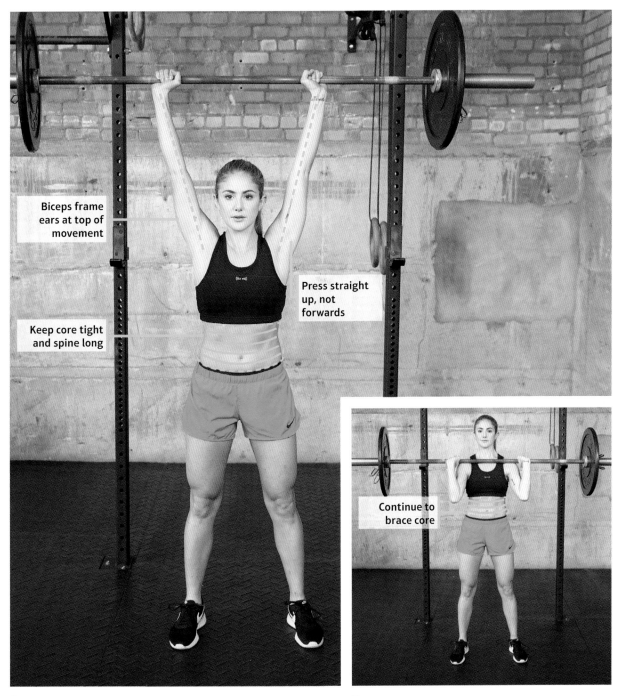

Biceps frame ears at top of movement

Press straight up, not forwards

Keep core tight and spine long

Continue to brace core

2 Exhale and use your shoulders to press the barbell straight up until your arms are fully extended. Keep your core tight to maintain stability without leaning forwards or backwards.

3 In a slow, controlled manner, lower the barbell to the starting position. That is one rep. Repeat for the number of reps given in your workout. Then re-rack the bar.

PULL-UP

There is nothing like a pull-up to make you feel strong. This exercise recruits your upper back to lift the weight of your entire body. For the full benefit, do not swing your legs, and push yourself to reach the top and bottom positions of the repetition each time.

EXERCISE PROFILE

Equipment
PULL-UP BAR

Primary muscle group
BACK

Secondary muscle group
SHOULDERS

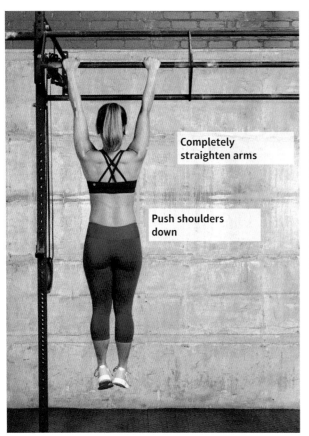

Completely straighten arms

Push shoulders down

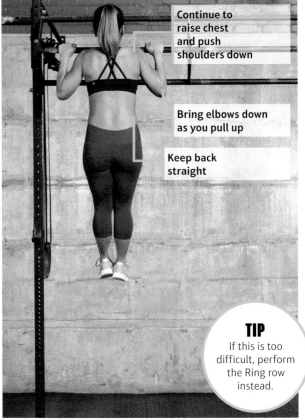

Continue to raise chest and push shoulders down

Bring elbows down as you pull up

Keep back straight

TIP
If this is too difficult, perform the Ring row instead.

1 Jump up to grab the bar. Place your hands shoulder-width apart, palms facing away from you, and grip tightly. Straighten your arms and let your body hang. Raise your chest.

2 Use your back to pull your body up until your chin is above the bar. Pause, then lower your body with control to the starting position. That is one rep. Repeat for the number of reps given in your workout.

CHIN-UP

Similar to the pull-up, the chin-up is a powerful strength movement, requiring you to lift the weight of your body. The underhand grip activates your biceps, making the movement slightly easier than a pull-up. Try not to short-change yourself by swinging and using momentum.

EXERCISE PROFILE

Equipment
PULL-UP BAR

Primary muscle groups
BACK, BICEPS

Secondary muscle groups
SHOULDERS, CHEST

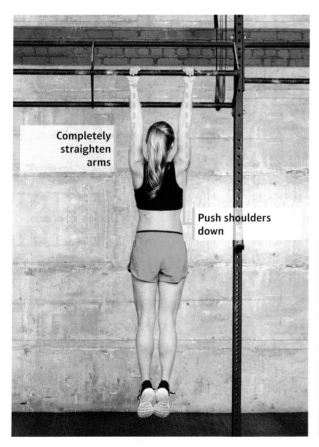

Completely straighten arms

Push shoulders down

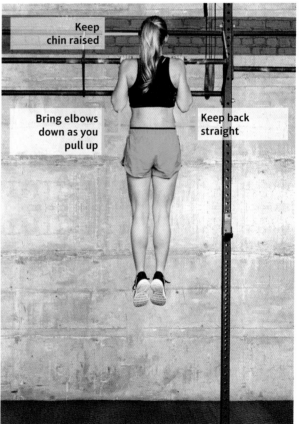

Keep chin raised

Bring elbows down as you pull up

Keep back straight

1 Jump up to grab the bar. Place your hands shoulder-width apart, palms facing towards you, and grip tightly. Straighten your arms and let your body hang. Raise your chest.

2 Use your back and biceps to pull your body up until your chin is above the bar. Pause, then lower your body with control to the starting position. That is one rep. Repeat for the number of reps given in your workout.

PUSH-UP

While it seems simple, the push-up is a very difficult and effective bodyweight move to have in your repertoire. In addition to building upper-body strength, it also improves shoulder mobility and works your core. The abs, obliques, and lower back are engaged to maintain stability throughout the movement.

EXERCISE PROFILE

Equipment
NONE

Primary muscle groups
CHEST, ABDOMINALS

Secondary muscle groups
SHOULDERS, TRICEPS

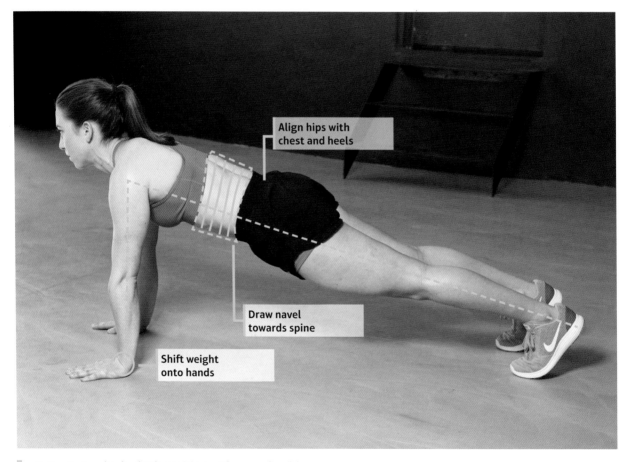

Align hips with chest and heels

Draw navel towards spine

Shift weight onto hands

1 Begin in a high plank position with your shoulders above your hands and your toes hip-width apart. Shift your weight forwards onto your hands and engage your core.

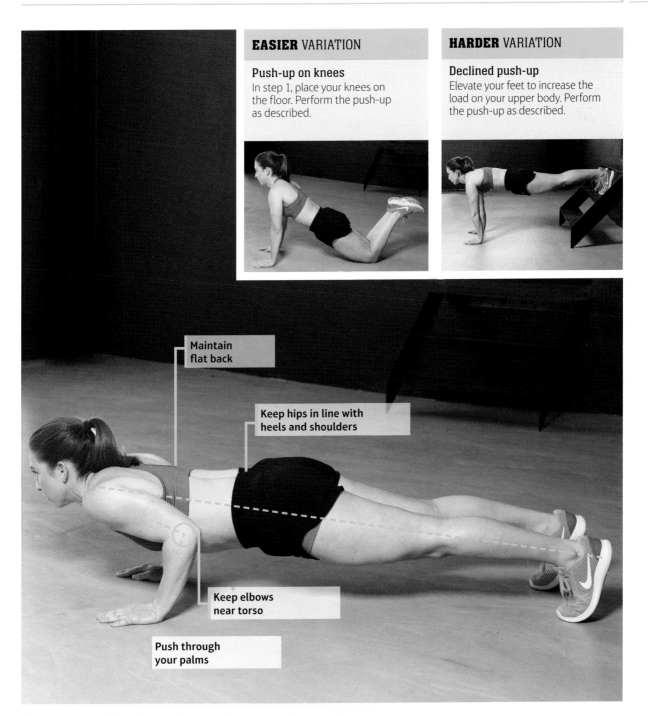

EASIER VARIATION

Push-up on knees
In step 1, place your knees on the floor. Perform the push-up as described.

HARDER VARIATION

Declined push-up
Elevate your feet to increase the load on your upper body. Perform the push-up as described.

Maintain flat back

Keep hips in line with heels and shoulders

Keep elbows near torso

Push through your palms

2 Inhale and bend your elbows to lower your chest until your elbows are bent to 90 degrees. Then exhale and push through your palms to return to the starting position. That is one rep. Repeat for the number of reps given in your workout.

T PUSH-UP

This advanced push-up variation is a fantastic way to build core strength and stability while also stretching your chest muscles and toning your upper back. The core rotation targets your obliques, leaving your entire body exhausted.

EXERCISE PROFILE

Equipment
NONE

Primary muscle groups
CHEST, CORE

Secondary muscle groups
SHOULDERS, TRICEPS, BACK

1 Begin in a high plank position with your shoulders above your hands and your toes wider than hip-width apart. Shift your weight forwards to your hands and engage your core.

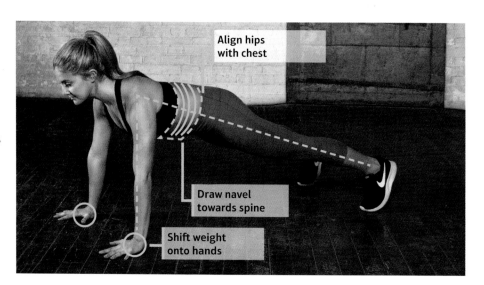

Align hips with chest

Draw navel towards spine

Shift weight onto hands

2 Inhale and bend your elbows to lower your chest until your elbows are bent to 90 degrees.

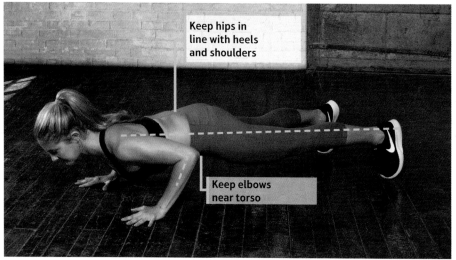

Keep hips in line with heels and shoulders

Keep elbows near torso

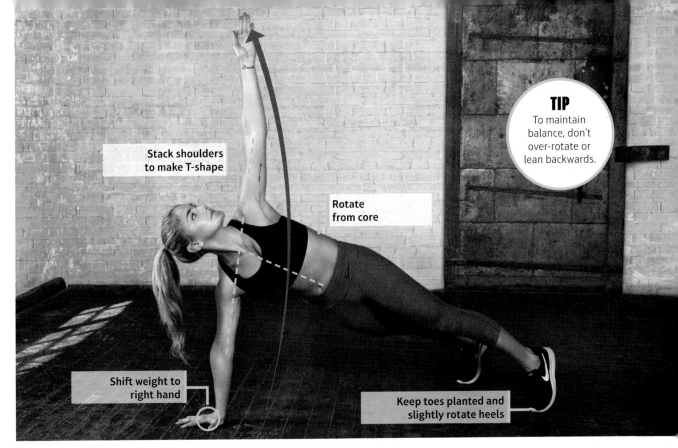

Stack shoulders
to make T-shape

Rotate
from core

TIP
To maintain
balance, don't
over-rotate or
lean backwards.

Shift weight to
right hand

Keep toes planted and
slightly rotate heels

3 Exhale and push through your palms to raise your body. In a continuous motion, fully extend your right arm, rotate your core to the left, and raise your left arm to the ceiling. Pause.

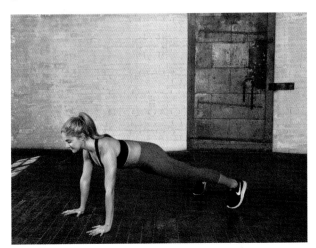

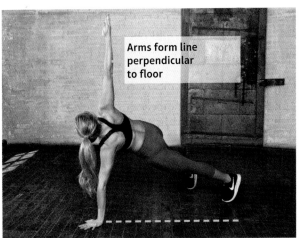

Arms form line
perpendicular
to floor

4 Return your left arm to the starting position. That is one rep.

5 Repeat the exercise, but this time raise your right arm. That is another rep. Alternate raising each arm for the number of reps given in your workout.

TRICEPS DIP

It is easy to neglect the backs of your arms, but this simple bodyweight exercise will make your triceps burn. The movement tones the muscles in the backs of your arms from shoulders to elbows, while also strengthening your core and chest.

EXERCISE PROFILE

Equipment
BENCH

Primary muscle group
TRICEPS

Secondary muscle groups
SHOULDERS, CORE, CHEST

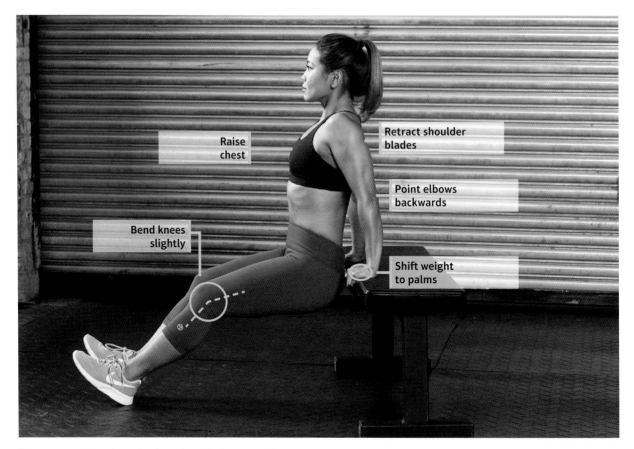

Raise chest

Retract shoulder blades

Point elbows backwards

Bend knees slightly

Shift weight to palms

1 Sit at the edge of a bench and place your hands shoulder-width apart by your hips. Shift your hips forwards off the bench and extend your legs. Shift your weight to the palms of your hands.

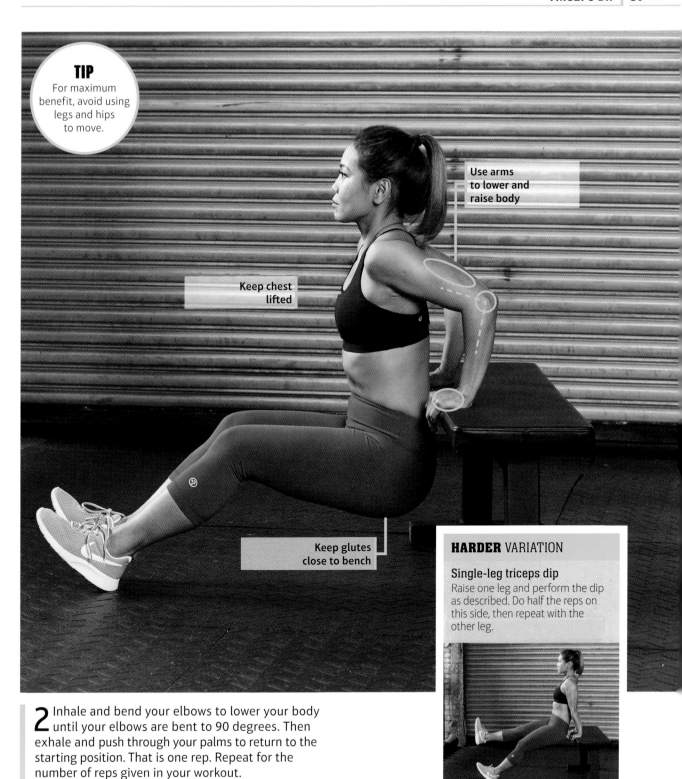

TIP
For maximum benefit, avoid using legs and hips to move.

Use arms to lower and raise body

Keep chest lifted

Keep glutes close to bench

HARDER VARIATION

Single-leg triceps dip
Raise one leg and perform the dip as described. Do half the reps on this side, then repeat with the other leg.

2 Inhale and bend your elbows to lower your body until your elbows are bent to 90 degrees. Then exhale and push through your palms to return to the starting position. That is one rep. Repeat for the number of reps given in your workout.

STANDING DUAL-DUMBBELL BICEPS CURL

A staple move for building upper-arm strength, the biceps curl will make your muscles firm and defined. Don't cheat yourself out of the benefits by swinging your arms. Maintain control for the entire movement.

EXERCISE PROFILE

Equipment
DUMBBELLS

Primary muscle group
BICEPS

Secondary muscle groups
SHOULDERS, DELTOIDS, CORE

1 Stand with your feet hip-width apart. Hold a dumbbell in each hand at your thighs, palms facing forwards. Engage your core and inhale.

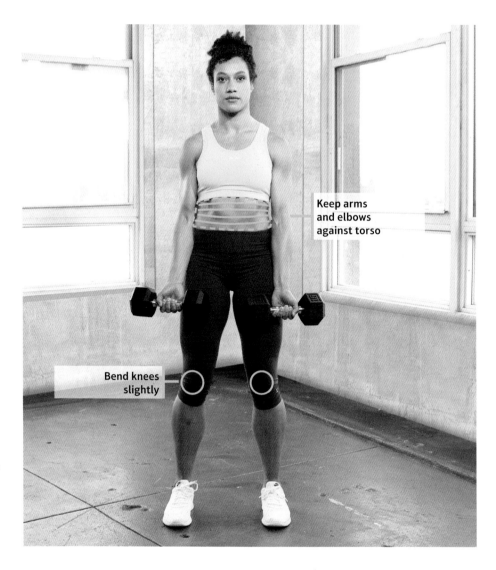

Keep arms and elbows against torso

Bend knees slightly

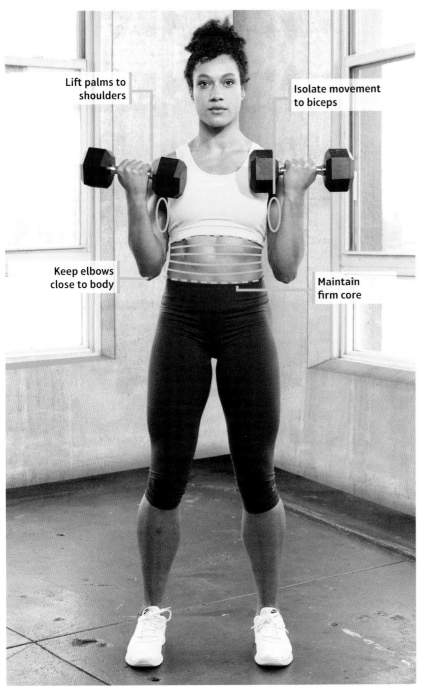

Lift palms to shoulders

Isolate movement to biceps

Keep elbows close to body

Maintain firm core

EASIER VARIATION

Hammer curl
In step 1, rotate your hands so your palms face each other, and perform the exercise as described.

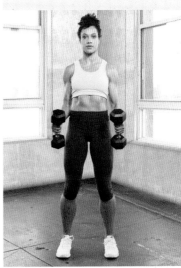

HARDER VARIATION

Squatting biceps curl
Perform the exercise from a deep squat position, starting with the weights near the floor. Stay in the squat the whole time.

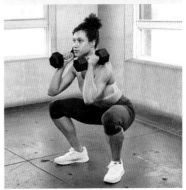

2 Exhale, and use your elbows as a hinge to curl the weights to your shoulders, keeping your arms close to your body. Then, in a controlled manner, lower your arms to the starting position. That is one rep. Repeat for the number of reps given in your workout.

BARBELL FRONT SQUAT

In this squat you hold the barbell in front of you, which is an effective way to develop leg power and overall strength. This variation of the squat works your core to keep your body stable and upright.

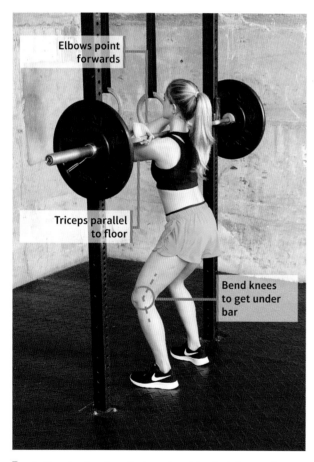

Elbows point forwards

Triceps parallel to floor

Bend knees to get under bar

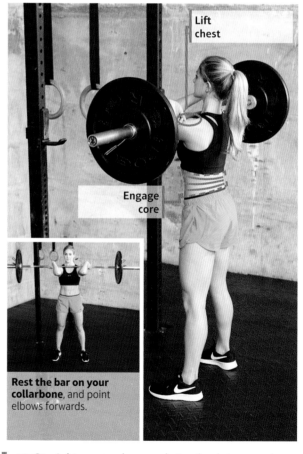

Lift chest

Engage core

Rest the bar on your collarbone, and point elbows forwards.

1 Set the bar just below shoulder height on the rack. Grasp the bar with your hands slightly wider than shoulder-width apart, palms facing up. Rest the bar on your collarbone.

2 Straighten your legs and step back to unrack the bar. Hold the weight on your collarbone (not your hands). Place your feet shoulder-width apart, and turn out your toes slightly.

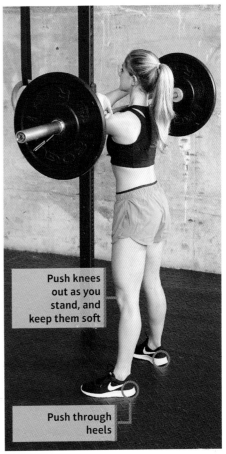

Push knees out as you stand, and keep them soft

Push through heels

4 Exhale and push through your heels to stand up. That is one rep. Repeat for the number of reps given in your workout. Then re-rack the bar.

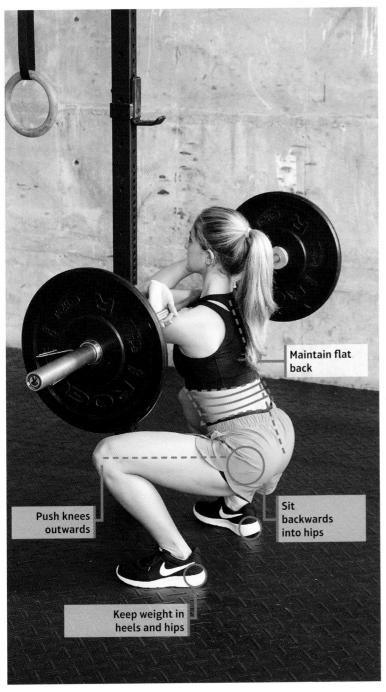

Maintain flat back

Push knees outwards

Sit backwards into hips

Keep weight in heels and hips

3 Brace your core, inhale, and push your hips back. Bend your knees and squat back until your thighs are parallel to the floor. Keep your glutes and core engaged and your weight in your heels.

BARBELL BACK SQUAT

This weighted squat is one of the best for developing leg power and overall strength, as well as total-body mobility. It is an energy-intensive movement that will boost your metabolism and burn body fat.

EXERCISE PROFILE

Equipment
BARBELL

Primary muscle group
QUADS

Secondary muscle groups
GLUTES, THIGHS, CORE

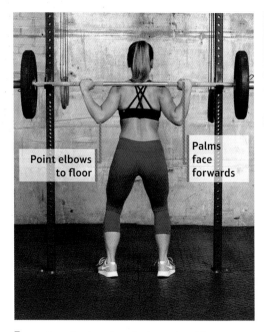

Point elbows to floor

Palms face forwards

1 Set the bar just below shoulder height on the rack. Step under the bar and position it on the back of your shoulders below your neck. Grasp the bar with your hands wider than shoulder-width apart.

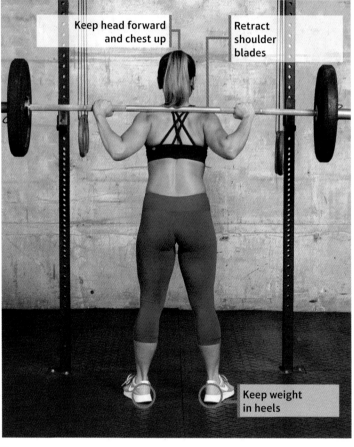

Keep head forward and chest up

Retract shoulder blades

Keep weight in heels

2 Straighten your legs and step back to unrack the bar. Hold the weight on your back (not your hands). Place your feet shoulder-width apart. Turn out your toes slightly.

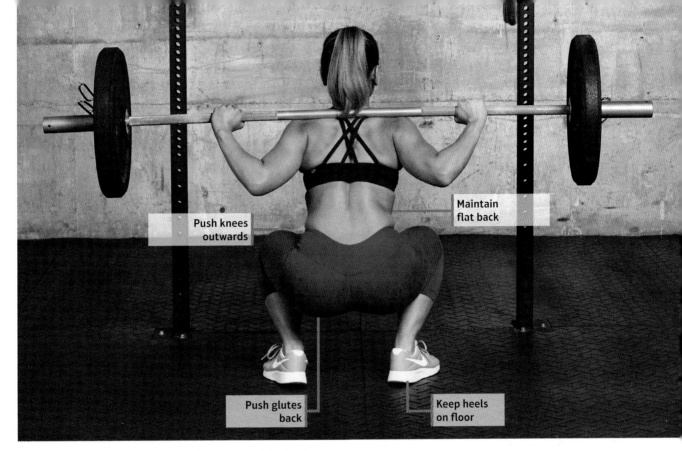

Push knees outwards

Maintain flat back

Push glutes back

Keep heels on floor

3 Brace your core, inhale, and push your hips back. Bend your knees and squat back until your thighs are parallel to the floor. Keep your glutes and core engaged throughout the movement.

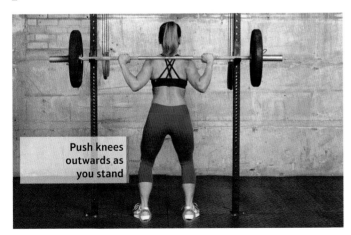

Push knees outwards as you stand

4 Exhale and push through your heels to stand up. That is one rep. Repeat for the number of reps given in your workout. Then re-rack the bar.

EASIER VARIATION

Bodyweight squat
Perform the squat as described, but without a barbell. Hold your hands together near your face.

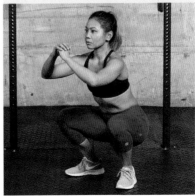

DUMBBELL
SUMO SQUAT

The wide open stance of this squat targets your hip adductors, the muscles that pull your thighs inwards. The movement also strengthens your glutes and thighs for toned, lean legs. The added resistance of the dumbbell maximizes the effect.

EXERCISE PROFILE

Equipment
DUMBBELL

Primary muscle groups
HIPS, GLUTES

Secondary muscle groups
QUADS, HAMSTRINGS, CORE

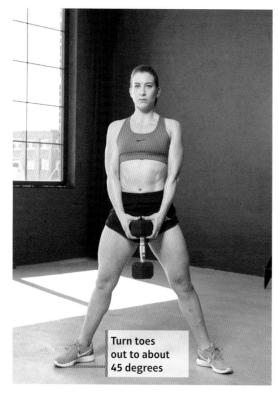

Turn toes out to about 45 degrees

1 Stand with your feet wide, and turn your toes outwards. Hold the top of a dumbbell between your legs, and let your arms hang straight down. Retract your shoulder blades.

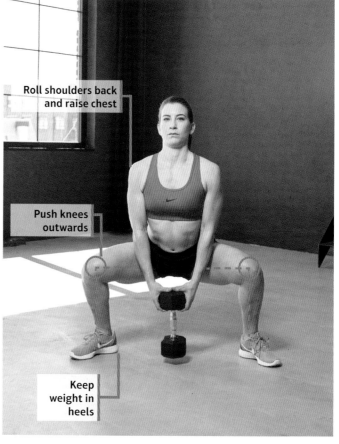

Roll shoulders back and raise chest

Push knees outwards

Keep weight in heels

2 Inhale, push your hips back, and bend your knees until your thighs are parallel to the floor. Let the dumbbell travel straight down. Keep your back flat.

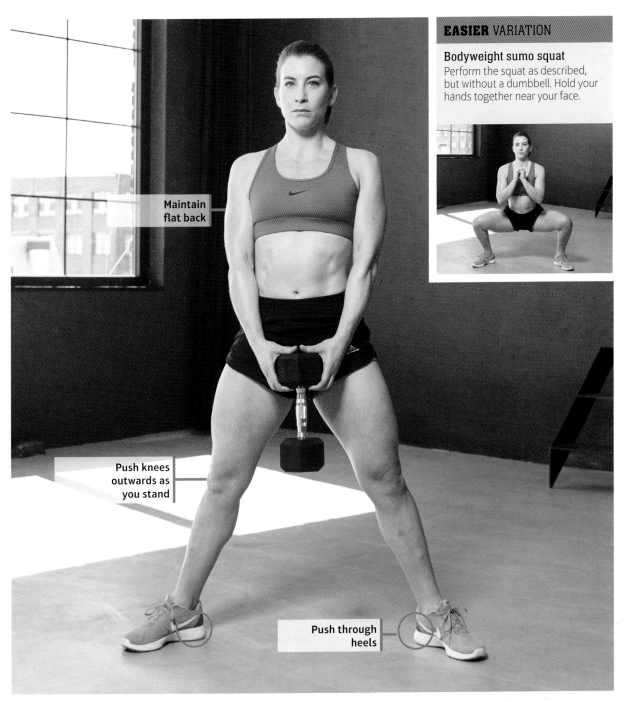

EASIER VARIATION

Bodyweight sumo squat
Perform the squat as described, but without a dumbbell. Hold your hands together near your face.

Maintain flat back

Push knees outwards as you stand

Push through heels

3 Exhale and push through your heels to stand up. That is one rep. Repeat for the number of reps given in your workout.

KETTLEBELL GOBLET SQUAT

The goblet squat is a great lower-body exercise for improving your squatting technique. The movement challenges your core, strengthens your legs, and improves spinal mobility.

EXERCISE PROFILE

Equipment
KETTLEBELL

Primary muscle groups
QUADS, HAMSTRINGS

Secondary muscle groups
GLUTES, SHOULDERS, CORE

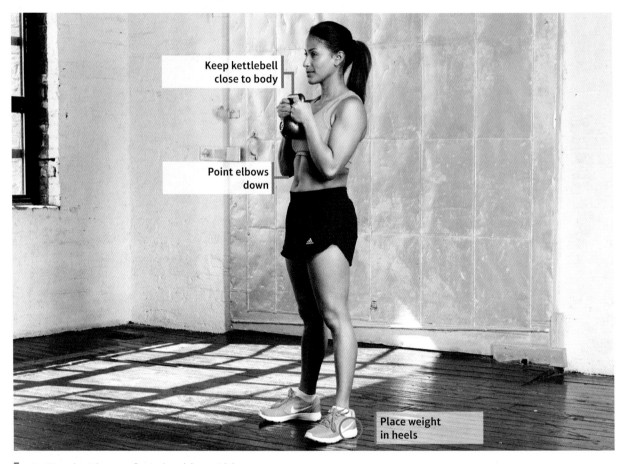

Keep kettlebell close to body

Point elbows down

Place weight in heels

1 Stand with your feet shoulder-width apart and turn out your toes slightly. Grasp a kettlebell with both hands and hold it close to your chest.

TIP
To keep feet stable, widen stance and press heels into floor.

Continue to hold kettlebell close to chest

Pull weight back into hips

Maintain upright torso

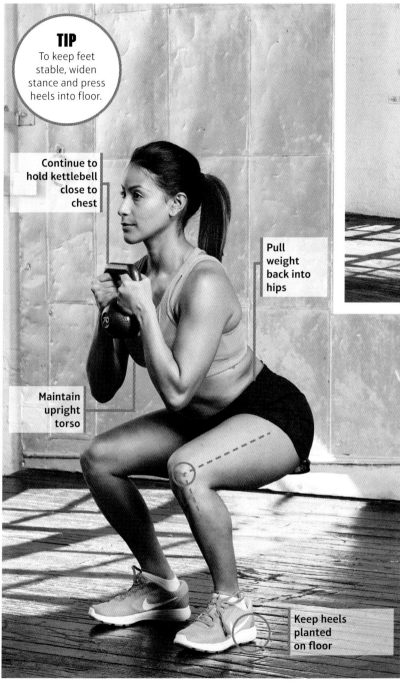

Keep heels planted on floor

2 Inhale, push your hips back, and bend your knees until your thighs are parallel to the floor.

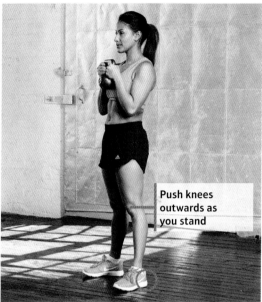

Push knees outwards as you stand

3 Exhale and push through your heels to stand up. That is one rep. Repeat for the number of reps given in your workout.

HARDER VARIATION

With thruster
As you stand up in step 3, press the kettlebell overhead. Then lower it back to your chest as you start the next rep.

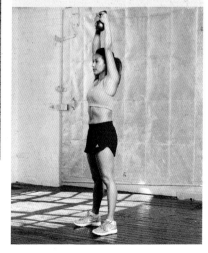

REAR-FOOT-ELEVATED
SPLIT SQUAT

Also known as an RFE or Bulgarian split squat, this exercise is one of the best for developing lower-body strength and power. It increases the flexibility of your hip flexors and challenges your core to maintain balance.

EXERCISE PROFILE

Equipment
DUMBBELLS, BENCH

Primary muscle groups
GLUTES, QUADS

Secondary muscle groups
HIPS, CORE

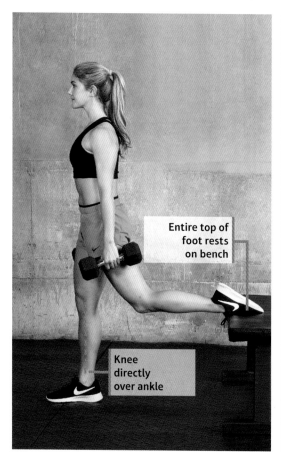

Entire top of foot rests on bench

Knee directly over ankle

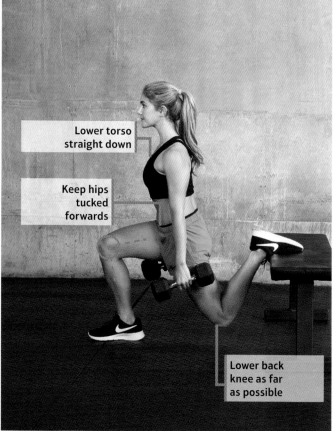

Lower torso straight down

Keep hips tucked forwards

Lower back knee as far as possible

1 Place the top of your left foot on a bench behind you, and plant your right foot firmly on the floor. Hold a dumbbell in each hand at your sides.

2 Inhale, bend both of your knees, and lower your left knee straight down until your right thigh is parallel to the floor.

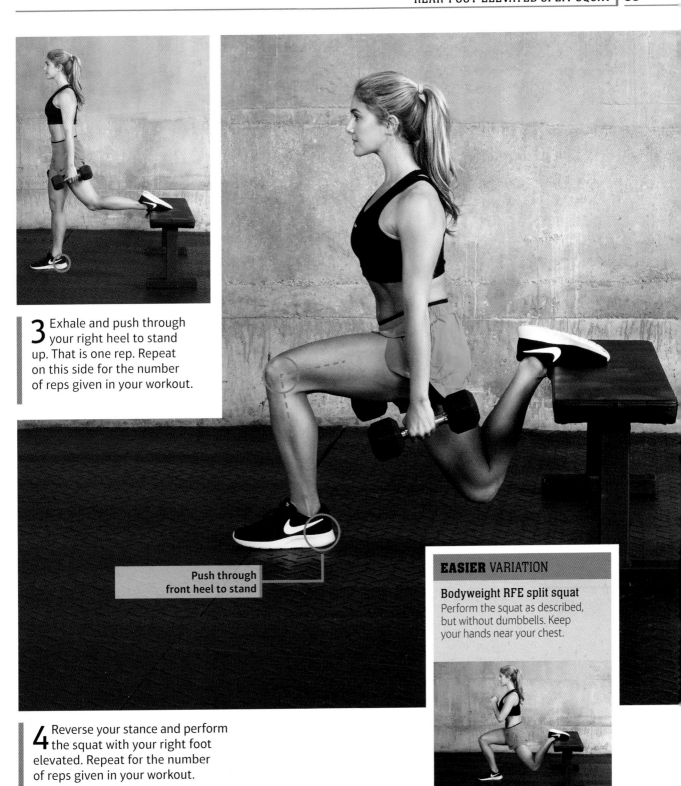

3 Exhale and push through your right heel to stand up. That is one rep. Repeat on this side for the number of reps given in your workout.

Push through front heel to stand

EASIER VARIATION

Bodyweight RFE split squat
Perform the squat as described, but without dumbbells. Keep your hands near your chest.

4 Reverse your stance and perform the squat with your right foot elevated. Repeat for the number of reps given in your workout.

BARBELL GOOD MORNING

This is a great movement for challenging your entire posterior chain (the back of your body). It is helpful for strengthening your lower back to prevent injury, as well as for firming your glutes.

EXERCISE PROFILE

Equipment
BARBELL

Primary muscle groups
GLUTES, HAMSTRINGS, LOWER BACK

Secondary muscle group
CORE

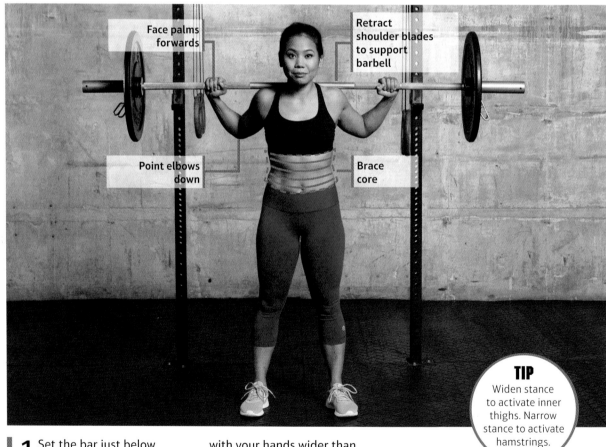

Face palms forwards

Retract shoulder blades to support barbell

Point elbows down

Brace core

TIP
Widen stance to activate inner thighs. Narrow stance to activate hamstrings.

1 Set the bar just below shoulder height on the rack. Step under the bar and position it on the back of your shoulders below your neck. Grasp the bar with your hands wider than shoulder-width apart. Straighten your legs and step forwards to unrack the bar. Place your feet shoulder-width apart.

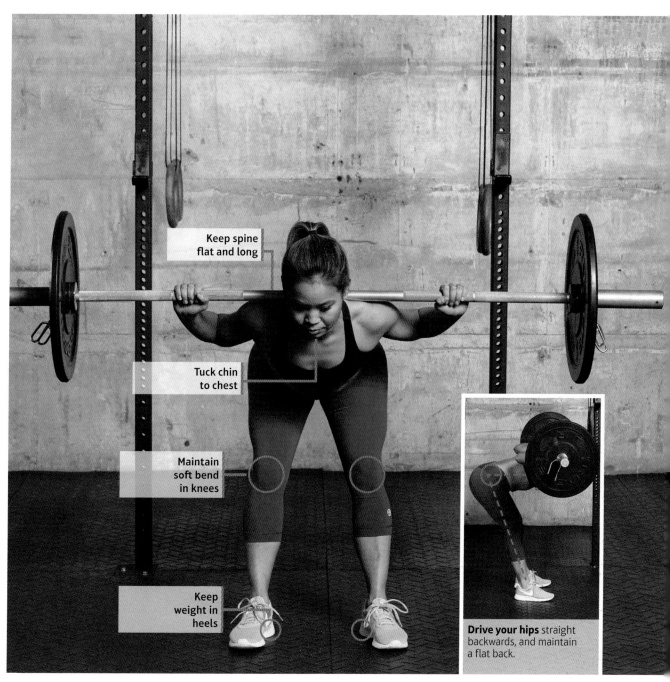

Keep spine flat and long

Tuck chin to chest

Maintain soft bend in knees

Keep weight in heels

Drive your hips straight backwards, and maintain a flat back.

2 Push your glutes back and hinge forwards at your hips to lower your chest until your torso is parallel to the floor. Then contract your hamstrings and glutes, and thrust your hips forwards to stand back up. That is one rep. Repeat for the number of reps given in your workout.

BARBELL GLUTE BRIDGE

Forming a bridge shape with your body is one of the best ways to isolate your gluteal muscles. Strong glutes look great and are incredibly important for overall power. This exercise conditions you for other barbell exercises and helps prevent lower back injury.

EXERCISE PROFILE

Equipment
BARBELL, BENCH

Primary muscle group
GLUTES

Secondary muscle groups
CORE, HAMSTRINGS

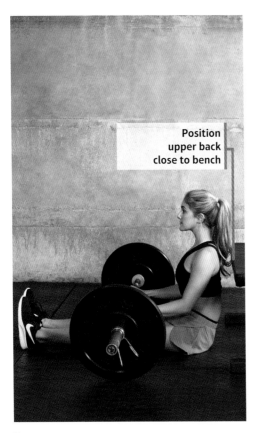

Position upper back close to bench

1 Sit on the floor in front of a bench with your legs extended. Place the bar over your thighs.

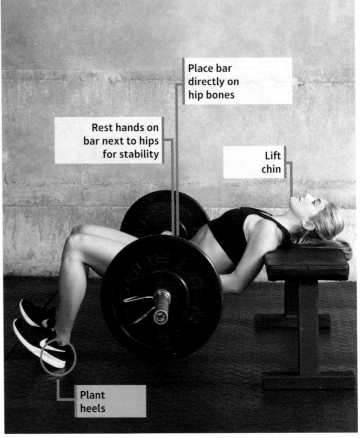

Place bar directly on hip bones

Rest hands on bar next to hips for stability

Lift chin

Plant heels

2 Get into position by lifting your hips and leaning back onto the bench. Rest your shoulder blades on the bench, bend your knees, and plant your heels firmly on the floor. Position the bar over your hip joints. Inhale.

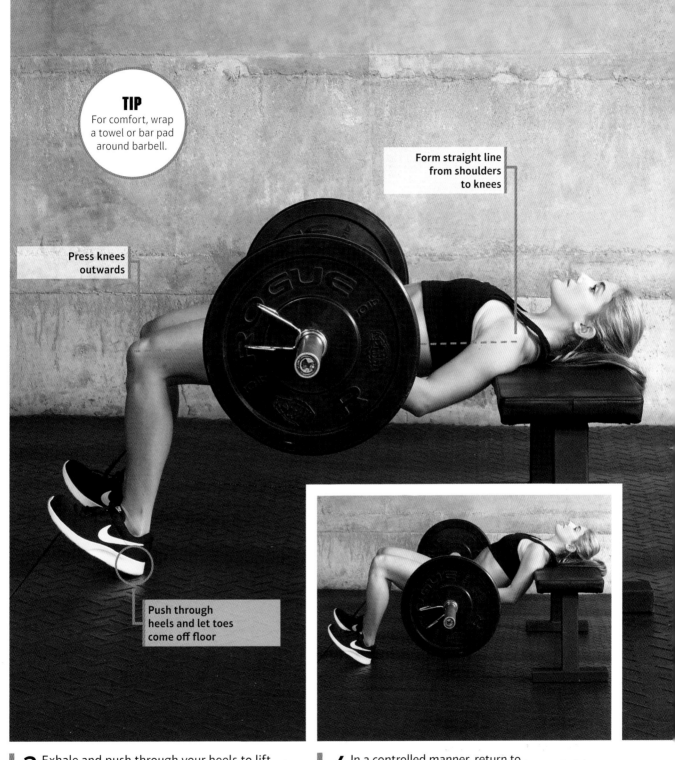

TIP
For comfort, wrap a towel or bar pad around barbell.

Form straight line from shoulders to knees

Press knees outwards

Push through heels and let toes come off floor

3 Exhale and push through your heels to lift your hips towards the ceiling, forming a straight line from your knees to your shoulders. Squeeze your glutes at the top of the movement.

4 In a controlled manner, return to the step 2 position. That is one rep. Repeat for the number of reps given in your workout.

DUMBBELL WALKING LUNGE

This is a basic lunge with a boost – you combine each rep in a fluid sequence as you walk forwards across the floor. It works all your leg muscles while also acting as a great stretch for the hip flexors. Your core activates to help keep you balanced.

EXERCISE PROFILE

Equipment
DUMBBELLS

Primary muscle groups
THIGHS, GLUTES

Secondary muscle groups
CORE, HIPS

CAUTION

Avoid this exercise if you have knee issues; stick to reverse lunges instead.

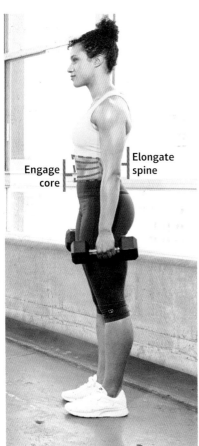

Engage core

Elongate spine

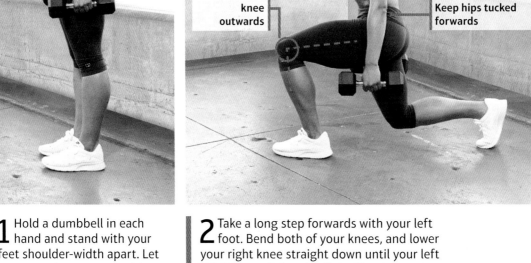

Lower torso straight down

Retract shoulder blades

Push knee outwards

Keep hips tucked forwards

1 Hold a dumbbell in each hand and stand with your feet shoulder-width apart. Let your arms hang at your sides.

2 Take a long step forwards with your left foot. Bend both of your knees, and lower your right knee straight down until your left thigh is parallel to the floor. That is one step.

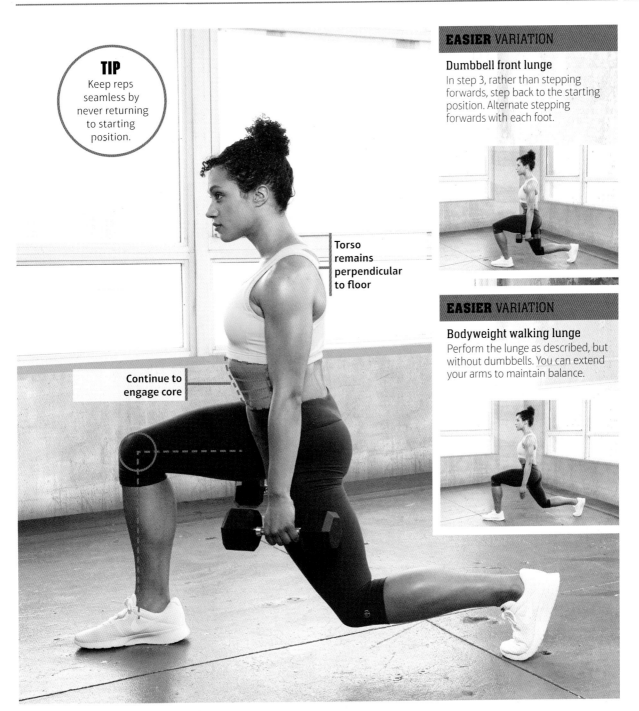

TIP
Keep reps seamless by never returning to starting position.

Torso remains perpendicular to floor

Continue to engage core

EASIER VARIATION

Dumbbell front lunge
In step 3, rather than stepping forwards, step back to the starting position. Alternate stepping forwards with each foot.

EASIER VARIATION

Bodyweight walking lunge
Perform the lunge as described, but without dumbbells. You can extend your arms to maintain balance.

3 Push through your left heel to stand up. Immediately take a long step forwards with your right foot. Bend your knees until your right thigh is parallel to the floor. That is another step. Continue lunging forwards for the number of steps given in your workout.

DUMBBELL REVERSE LUNGE

Performing lunges in reverse tones your legs while placing minimal stress on your knee joints compared to squats and forward lunges. Dumbbells increase the burn and challenge your balance.

EXERCISE PROFILE

Equipment
DUMBBELLS

Primary muscle groups
QUADS, GLUTES

Secondary muscle groups
LEGS, CORE

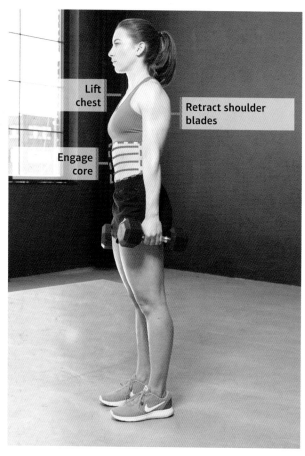

Lift chest

Retract shoulder blades

Engage core

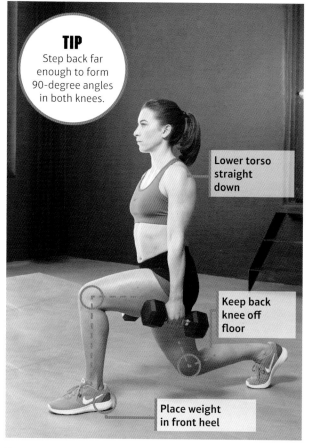

TIP
Step back far enough to form 90-degree angles in both knees.

Lower torso straight down

Keep back knee off floor

Place weight in front heel

1 Stand with your feet shoulder-width apart. Hold a dumbbell in each hand, and let your arms hang at your sides.

2 Take a long step back with your right foot. Bend both knees, and lower your right knee straight down until your left thigh is parallel to the floor.

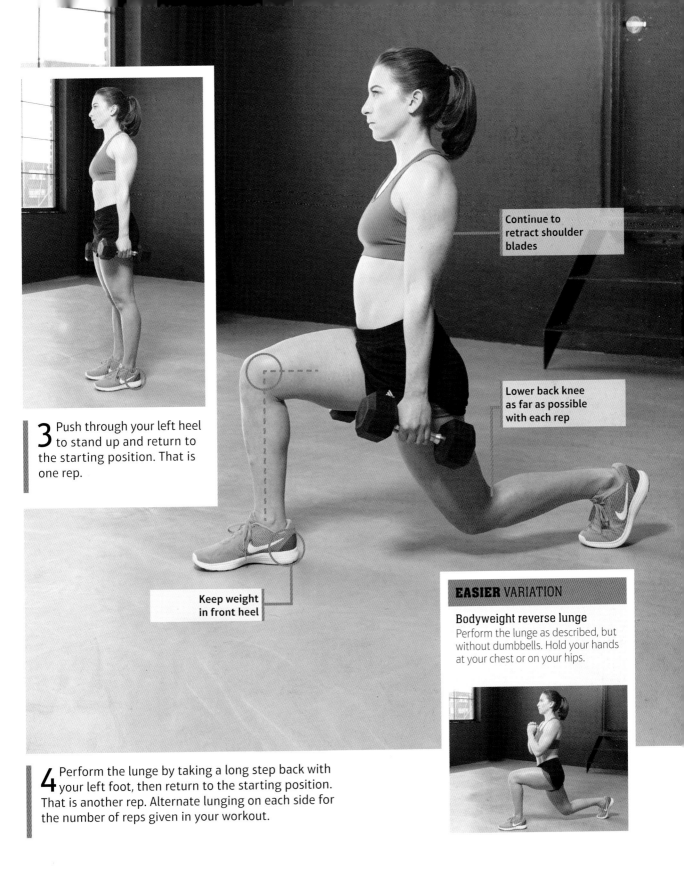

Continue to
retract shoulder
blades

Lower back knee
as far as possible
with each rep

3 Push through your left heel
to stand up and return to
the starting position. That is
one rep.

Keep weight
in front heel

EASIER VARIATION

Bodyweight reverse lunge
Perform the lunge as described, but
without dumbbells. Hold your hands
at your chest or on your hips.

4 Perform the lunge by taking a long step back with
your left foot, then return to the starting position.
That is another rep. Alternate lunging on each side for
the number of reps given in your workout.

DUMBBELL LATERAL LUNGE

Lunging from side to side ensures that your range of motion extends to all planes of movement. This exercise develops the muscles of your lower body and challenges your balance. The wide step firms and tones your glutes.

EXERCISE PROFILE

Equipment
DUMBBELLS

Primary muscle group
GLUTES

Secondary muscle groups
QUADS, HIPS, CORE

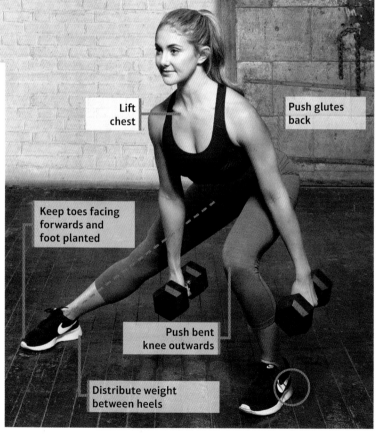

Lift chest

Push glutes back

Keep toes facing forwards and foot planted

Push bent knee outwards

Distribute weight between heels

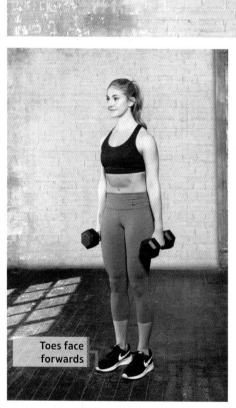

Toes face forwards

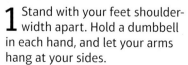

1 Stand with your feet shoulder-width apart. Hold a dumbbell in each hand, and let your arms hang at your sides.

2 Inhale and take a wide step to your left. Bend your left knee and sit your hips back until your left thigh is nearly parallel to the floor. Keep your right leg straight and let the weights move down to frame your bent knee.

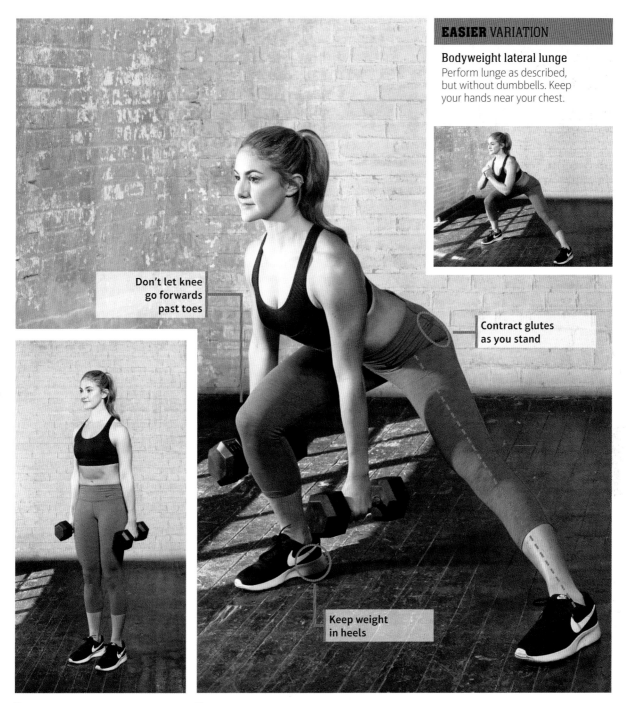

EASIER VARIATION

Bodyweight lateral lunge
Perform lunge as described, but without dumbbells. Keep your hands near your chest.

Don't let knee go forwards past toes

Contract glutes as you stand

Keep weight in heels

3 Exhale and push through your left heel to return to the starting position. That is one rep.

4 Perform the lunge to your right. That is another rep. Continue lunging, either alternating or staying on the same side for the number of reps given, according to your workout.

DUMBBELL STEP-UP

Stepping up onto a box is a multi-joint functional movement that develops strength in the lower body and challenges core stability and balance. It translates to more efficient movement in sport and daily life. The higher the box, the harder it is.

EXERCISE PROFILE

Equipment
DUMBBELLS, BOX

Primary muscle groups
QUADS, GLUTES

Secondary muscle groups
HAMSTRINGS, HIPS, CALVES, CORE

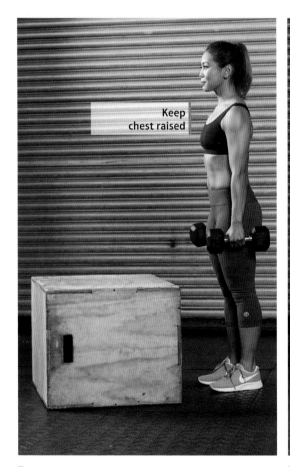

Keep chest raised

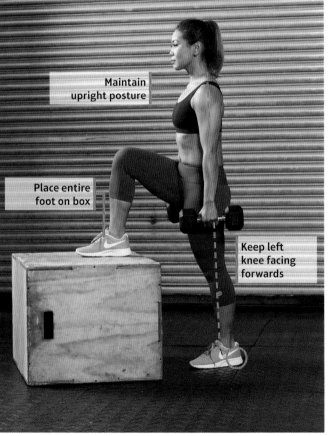

Maintain upright posture

Place entire foot on box

Keep left knee facing forwards

1 Stand behind a box or flat bench with your feet shoulder-width apart. Hold a dumbbell in each hand, and let your arms hang at your sides.

2 Bend your right knee and place your right foot fully on the box. Keep your left leg firmly planted on the floor.

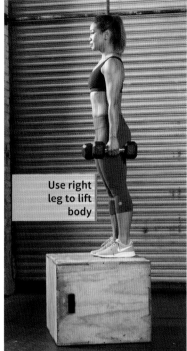

Use right leg to lift body

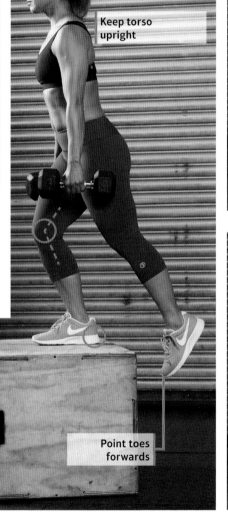

Keep torso upright

Point toes forwards

3 Push through your right heel to fully straighten your right leg and stand up. Place your left foot on the box, but do not use your left leg to push off the floor.

4 Carefully bend your right knee and place your left foot back on the floor to step down. Follow with your right foot to return to the starting position. That is one rep. Repeat the exercise with this leg for the number of reps given in your workout.

EASIER VARIATION

Bodyweight step-up
Perform the exercise as described, but without dumbbells. Let your arms hang at your sides.

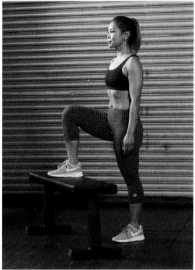

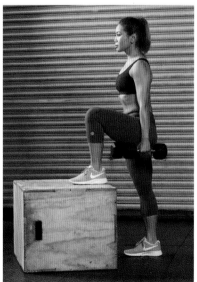

5 Perform the exercise with your left leg. That is another rep. Repeat with this leg for the number of reps given in your workout.

CONVENTIONAL BARBELL DEADLIFT

This deadlift increases total-body strength and develops lower-body power. It is also entirely functional, meaning the movement trains you for real-life applications that involve lifting heavy objects off the ground.

EXERCISE PROFILE

Equipment
BARBELL

Primary muscle groups
GLUTES, HAMSTRINGS

Secondary muscle groups
CORE, BACK

CAUTION

To protect your lower back, keep your core engaged throughout the exercise.

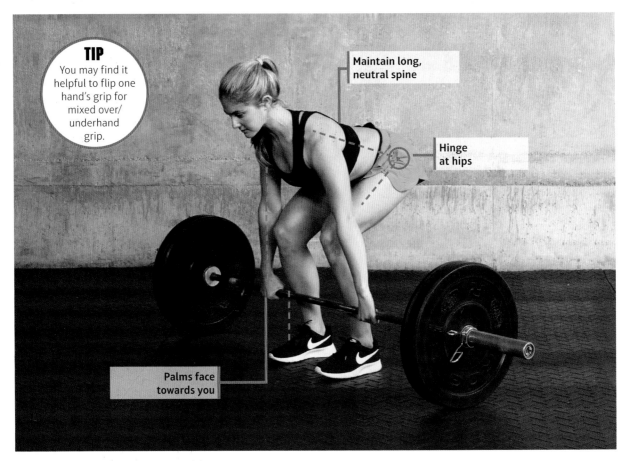

TIP
You may find it helpful to flip one hand's grip for mixed over/underhand grip.

Maintain long, neutral spine

Hinge at hips

Palms face towards you

1 Place your feet under the bar, shoulder-width apart, so the bar grazes your shins. Grip the barbell so your forearms touch the outsides of your thighs. Hinge forwards at the hips and push your glutes back. Align your shoulders over the bar and retract your shoulder blades to activate your back. Inhale.

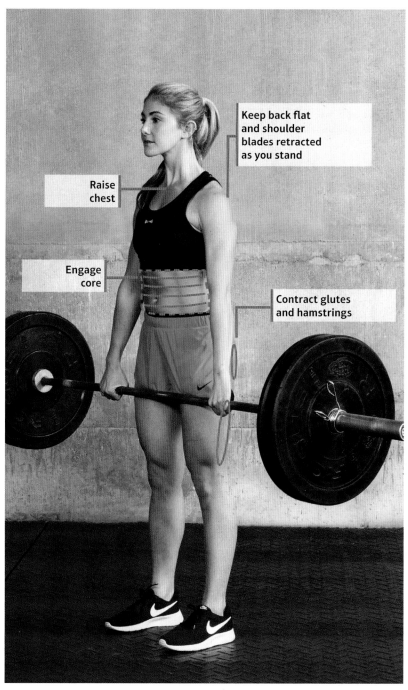

Raise chest

Keep back flat and shoulder blades retracted as you stand

Engage core

Contract glutes and hamstrings

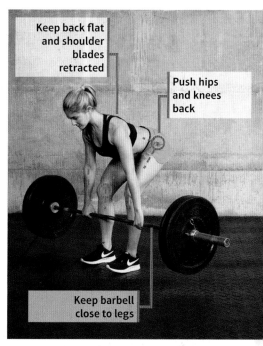

Keep back flat and shoulder blades retracted

Push hips and knees back

Keep barbell close to legs

3 Push your hips back. Bend your knees to return the barbell to the floor, keeping your shoulders over the bar the entire time. That is one rep. Repeat for the number of reps given in your workout.

EASIER VARIATION

Kettlebell deadlift
Perform the exercise as described, but with a kettlebell. Place the weight between your ankles and hold the handle firmly with both hands.

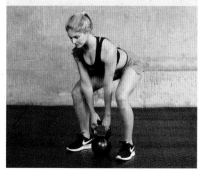

2 Exhale, push through your heels, and use your glutes and hamstrings to stand up. Keep the barbell close to your body and stack your shoulders directly over your hips.

DUMBBELL ROMANIAN DEADLIFT

Also known as the RDL, this is one of the best exercises for targeting your hamstrings and glutes while engaging your core. The weight of the dumbbells and the deep range of motion work to strengthen lower-body muscles.

EXERCISE PROFILE

Equipment
DUMBBELLS

Primary muscle groups
HAMSTRINGS, GLUTES

Secondary muscle groups
CORE, CALVES

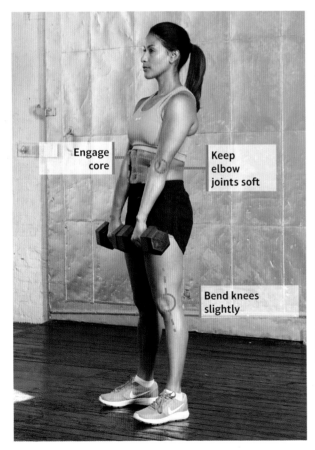

Engage core

Keep elbow joints soft

Bend knees slightly

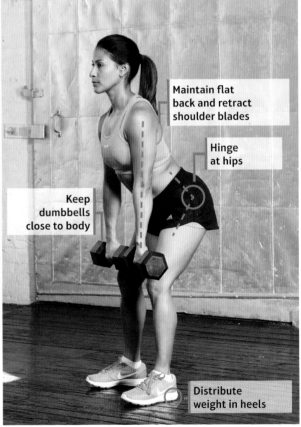

Maintain flat back and retract shoulder blades

Hinge at hips

Keep dumbbells close to body

Distribute weight in heels

1 Stand with your feet shoulder-width apart. Hold a dumbbell in each hand with your arms in front of you, palms facing your thighs. Bend your knees slightly. Elongate your spine.

2 Slowly hinge forwards at the hips and push your glutes back, letting your knees bend slightly. Keep your shoulders aligned directly over the dumbbells.

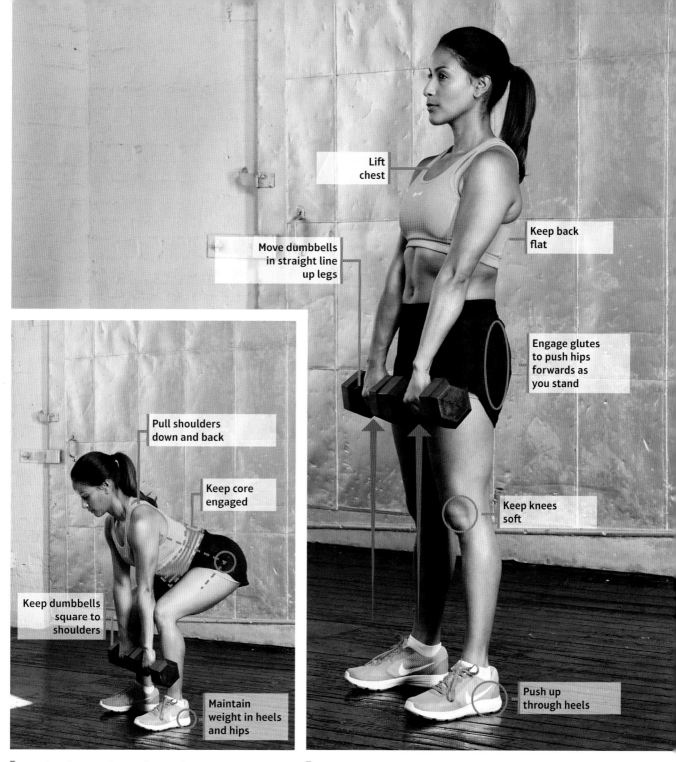

Lift chest

Keep back flat

Move dumbbells in straight line up legs

Engage glutes to push hips forwards as you stand

Pull shoulders down and back

Keep core engaged

Keep knees soft

Keep dumbbells square to shoulders

Maintain weight in heels and hips

Push up through heels

3 Continue to hinge forwards at your hips until the dumbbells reach the middle of your shins. Keep your back long and flat.

4 Push through your heels, engage your glutes, and straighten your legs and hips to return to the starting position. That is one rep. Repeat for the number of reps given in your workout.

KETTLEBELL SINGLE-LEG DEADLIFT

Working one side of your body at a time is necessary for increasing your overall stability and balance. Standing on one leg challenges your core, isolates your glutes, and activates your entire posterior chain.

EXERCISE PROFILE

Equipment
KETTLEBELL

Primary muscle groups
GLUTES, HAMSTRINGS, QUADS

Secondary muscle groups
CORE, HIPS

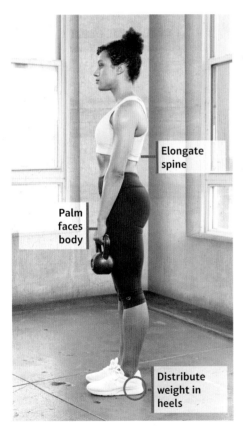

Elongate spine

Palm faces body

Distribute weight in heels

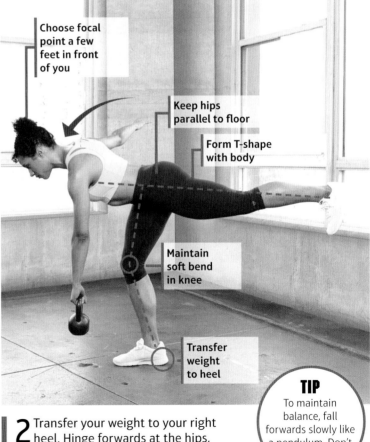

Choose focal point a few feet in front of you

Keep hips parallel to floor

Form T-shape with body

Maintain soft bend in knee

Transfer weight to heel

1 Stand with your feet hip-width apart. Hold the handle of a kettlebell in your left hand at your left thigh.

2 Transfer your weight to your right heel. Hinge forwards at the hips, bring your torso forwards, and extend your left leg back until your torso is parallel to the floor. Suspend the kettlebell under your shoulder.

TIP
To maintain balance, fall forwards slowly like a pendulum. Don't kick leg back.

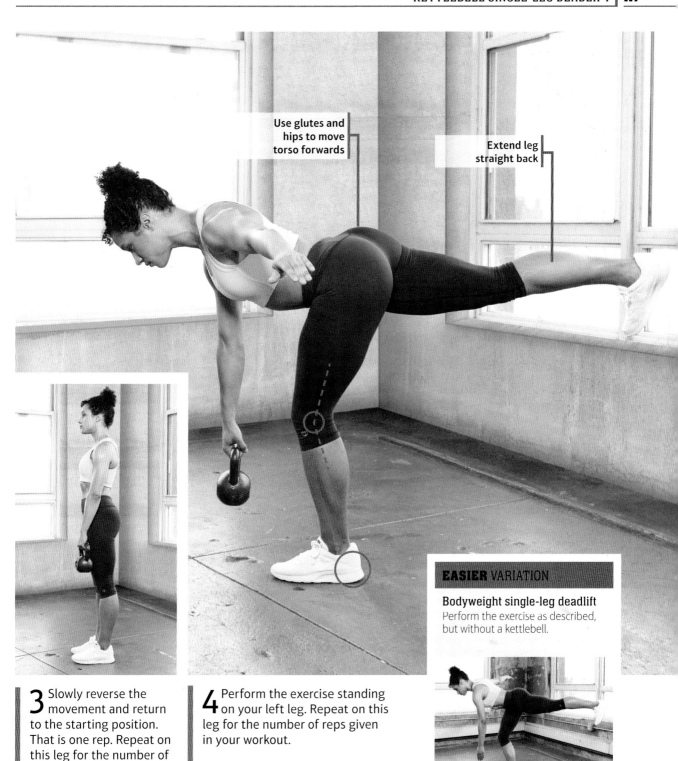

Use glutes and hips to move torso forwards

Extend leg straight back

EASIER VARIATION

Bodyweight single-leg deadlift
Perform the exercise as described, but without a kettlebell.

3 Slowly reverse the movement and return to the starting position. That is one rep. Repeat on this leg for the number of reps given in your workout.

4 Perform the exercise standing on your left leg. Repeat on this leg for the number of reps given in your workout.

BURPEE

Test your endurance and condition your whole body with this bodyweight exercise. Burpees combine explosive plyometric movements with the strength-building power of push-ups to leave you dripping in sweat. They are very challenging and highly effective at burning fat.

EXERCISE PROFILE

Equipment
NONE

Primary muscle groups
LEGS, CORE

Secondary muscle groups
SHOULDERS, ARMS, CHEST

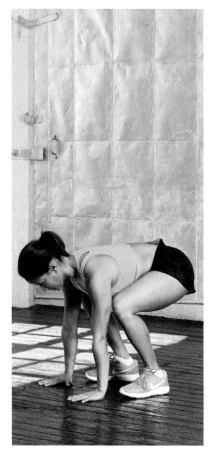

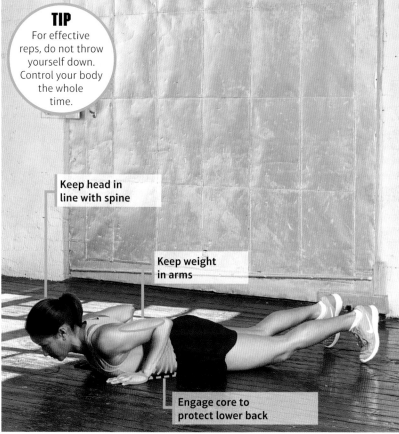

TIP
For effective reps, do not throw yourself down. Control your body the whole time.

Keep head in line with spine

Keep weight in arms

Engage core to protect lower back

1 Stand with your feet hip-width apart. Crouch down and place your hands on the floor in front of your toes.

2 Quickly jump your feet back to a high plank position, then lower your body to the floor for a push-up.

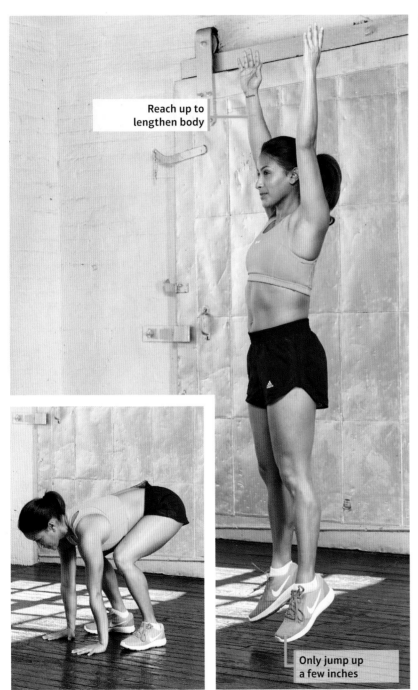

Reach up to lengthen body

Only jump up a few inches

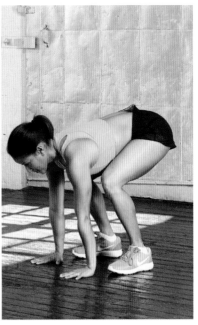

5 Return to the starting position. Repeat for the number of reps given in your workout.

EASIER VARIATION

Jump back burpee
In step 2, jump your feet back to a high plank, but do not lower your body for a push-up. Then proceed to step 3.

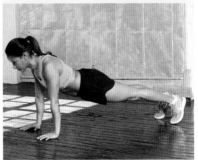

3 Extend your arms out of the push-up, and immediately hop your feet back towards your hands.

4 Quickly jump up and reach your hands over your head. That is one rep.

PLYO PUSH-UP

Adding an explosive element to the classic push-up activates the muscle fibres that are responsible for powerful muscle movements. This increases overall calorie burn, strength, and muscle growth.

EXERCISE PROFILE

Equipment
NONE

Primary muscle groups
CHEST, SHOULDERS

Secondary muscle groups
CORE, TRICEPS, BACK

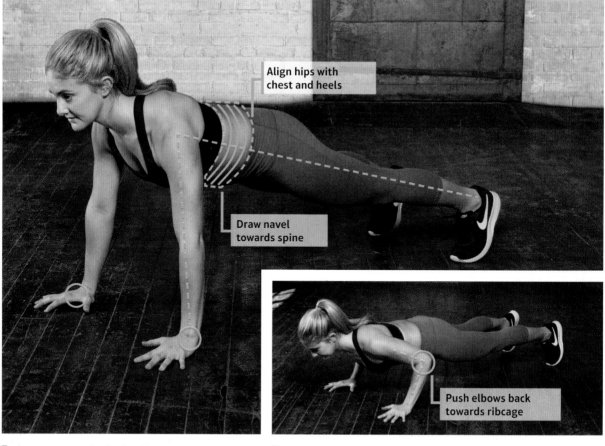

Align hips with chest and heels

Draw navel towards spine

Push elbows back towards ribcage

1 Begin in a high plank position with your shoulders above your hands and your toes hip-width apart. Shift your weight forward to your hands and engage your core.

2 Inhale and bend your elbows to lower your chest towards the floor until your elbows are bent to 90 degrees.

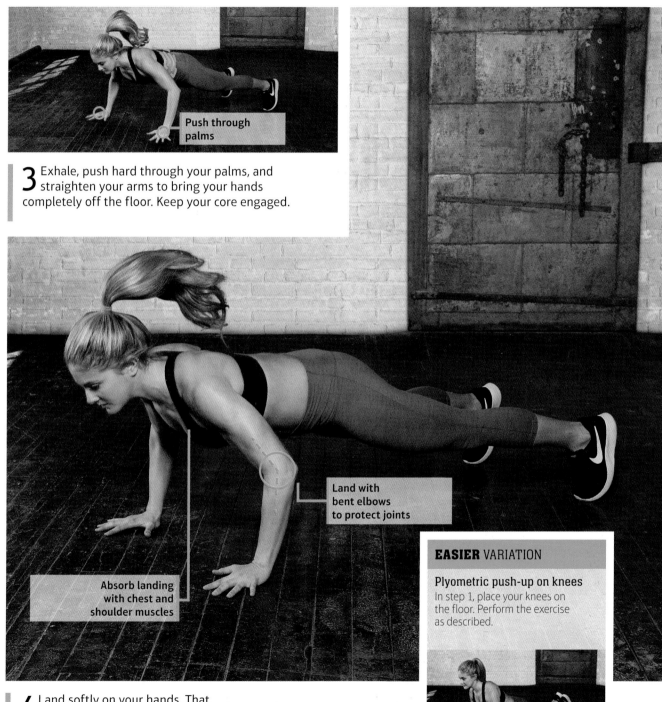

Push through palms

3 Exhale, push hard through your palms, and straighten your arms to bring your hands completely off the floor. Keep your core engaged.

Land with bent elbows to protect joints

Absorb landing with chest and shoulder muscles

EASIER VARIATION

Plyometric push-up on knees
In step 1, place your knees on the floor. Perform the exercise as described.

4 Land softly on your hands. That is one rep. Immediately transition into the next push-up. Repeat for the number of reps given in your workout.

BOX JUMP

Plyometric exercises – those involving jumping – are a great test of explosive power, athleticism, and strength. This common plyometric exercise develops lower-body power, increases your heart rate, and helps your body build muscle at a rapid pace.

EXERCISE PROFILE

Equipment
BOX

Primary muscle groups
HIPS, GLUTES, HAMSTRINGS

Secondary muscle groups
CALVES, CORE

CAUTION

Step down from the box to avoid ankle stress. Don't jump.

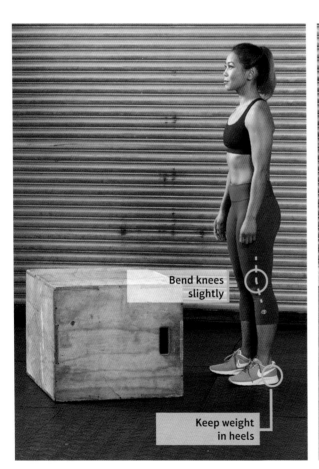

Bend knees slightly

Keep weight in heels

1 Stand behind a box or flat bench with your feet shoulder-width apart. Rest your arms at your sides.

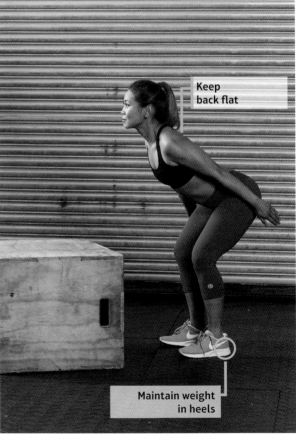

Keep back flat

Maintain weight in heels

2 Push your hips back and bend your knees to enter into a slight squat. Swing your arms behind you for momentum.

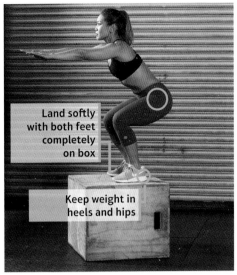

4 Land with your feet flat on the box and your weight in your heels. Bend your knees to absorb the landing.

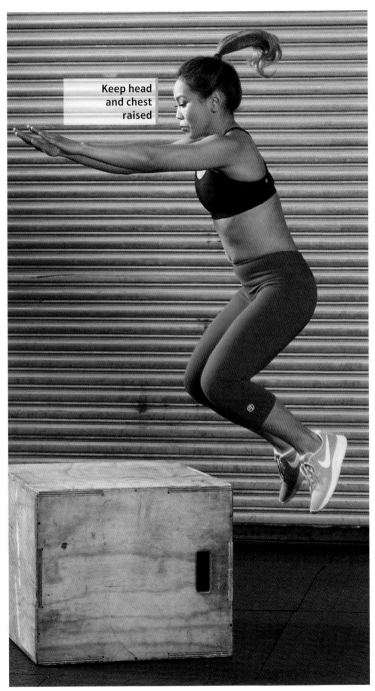

Keep head and chest raised

Land softly with both feet completely on box

Keep weight in heels and hips

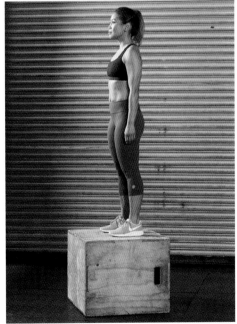

3 Push through your heels and jump up onto the box, swinging your arms forwards.

5 Stand up, then carefully step back down to the starting position. That is one rep. Repeat for the number of reps given in your workout.

JUMP LUNGE

Adding a jump to any movement instantly increases the intensity and burns more calories. The jump lunge fires up all the muscles in your legs while engaging your core. This exercise makes you stronger and improves your stability and balance.

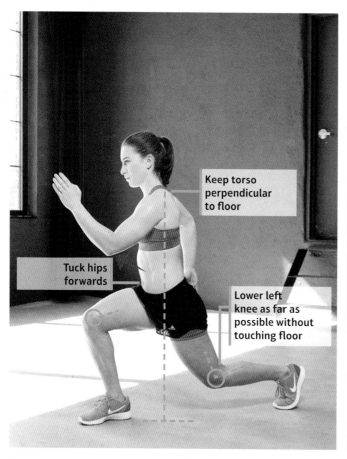

Keep torso perpendicular to floor

Tuck hips forwards

Lower left knee as far as possible without touching floor

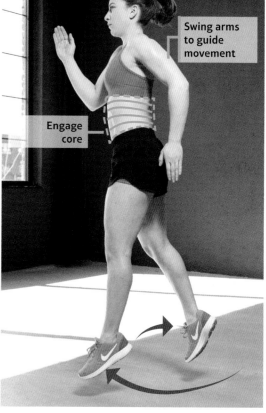

Swing arms to guide movement

Engage core

1 Begin in a lunge with your left foot far back. Bend your knees to 90 degrees, and rise up onto the ball of your left foot. Bend your elbows, draw your left arm forwards, and pull your right arm back.

2 Vigorously push through your feet and jump up as high as you can. Switch your arm and leg positions in the air.

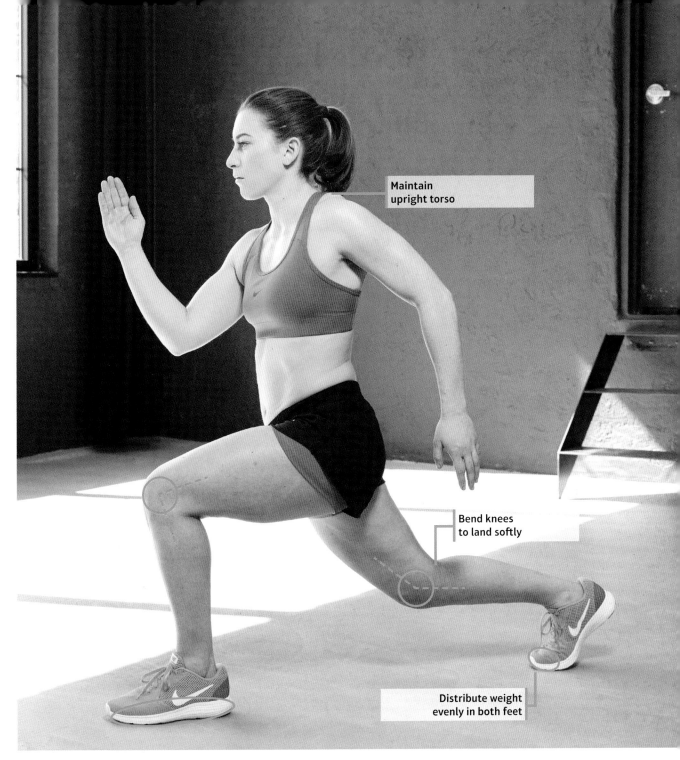

Maintain upright torso

Bend knees to land softly

Distribute weight evenly in both feet

3 Land in a lunge with your left foot forward and your right foot back. That is one rep. Continue to jump and alternate lunging on each side for the number of reps given in your workout.

DUAL-KETTLEBELL PUSH PRESS

Considered a plyometric exercise for your upper body, this exercise develops explosive power and strength in your shoulders. Even though it isolates your arms, the entire body activates to push the kettlebells overhead.

EXERCISE PROFILE

Equipment
KETTLEBELLS

Primary muscle groups
SHOULDERS, BACK

Secondary muscle groups
CORE, BICEPS, HIPS

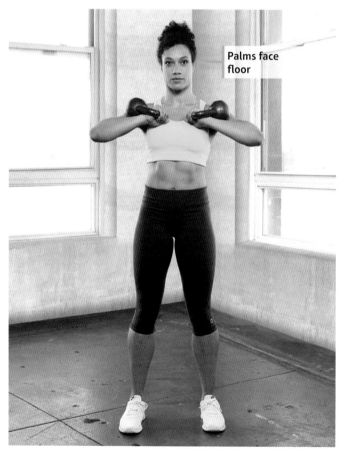

Palms face floor

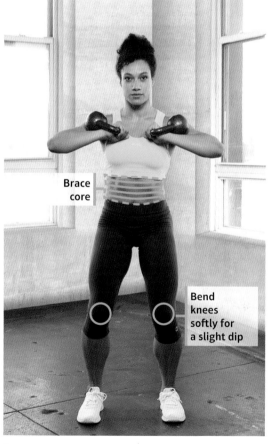

Brace core

Bend knees softly for a slight dip

1 Stand with your feet hip-width apart. Hold a kettlebell in each hand with the handles just below your collarbone. Rest the weights on your forearms and point your elbows out to the sides. Inhale.

2 Exhale and bend your knees slightly. Engage your core and retract your shoulder blades. Lengthen your torso.

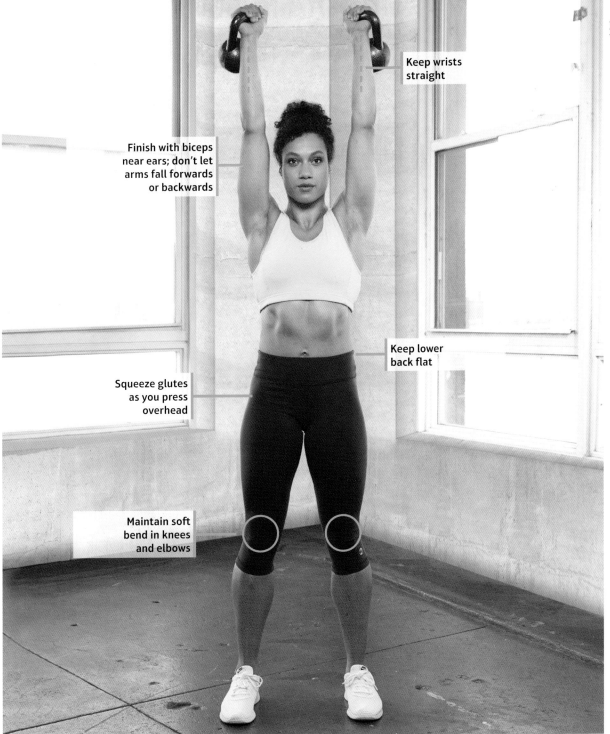

Keep wrists straight

Finish with biceps near ears; don't let arms fall forwards or backwards

Keep lower back flat

Squeeze glutes as you press overhead

Maintain soft bend in knees and elbows

3 Vigorously push through your heels, straighten your legs, and use your shoulders to press the kettlebells overhead, palms facing the ceiling. Then return to the starting position. That is one rep. Repeat for the number of reps given in your workout.

JUMP SQUAT

These plyometric squats tone your leg muscles and strengthen your core. Since they're effective and don't require equipment, jump squats are a perfect addition to any strength programme. They elevate your heart rate, burn lots of calories, and build muscles for speed and power.

EXERCISE PROFILE

Equipment
NONE

Primary muscle groups
GLUTES, QUADS

Secondary muscle groups
HAMSTRINGS, CALVES, CORE

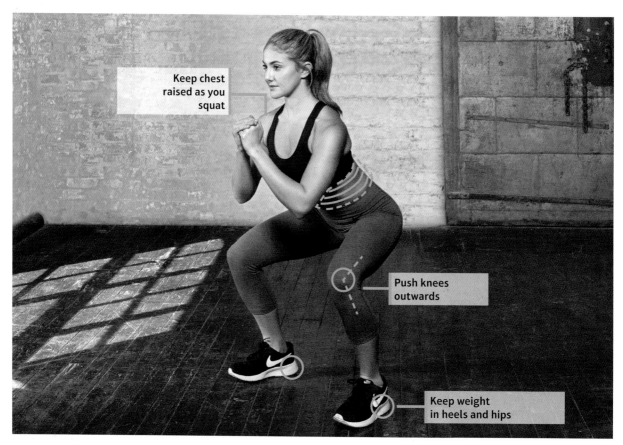

Keep chest raised as you squat

Push knees outwards

Keep weight in heels and hips

1 Stand with your feet shoulder-width apart and turn your toes slightly outwards. Inhale, push your hips back, and bend your knees until your thighs are roughly parallel to the floor. Clasp your hands at your chest and keep your core engaged.

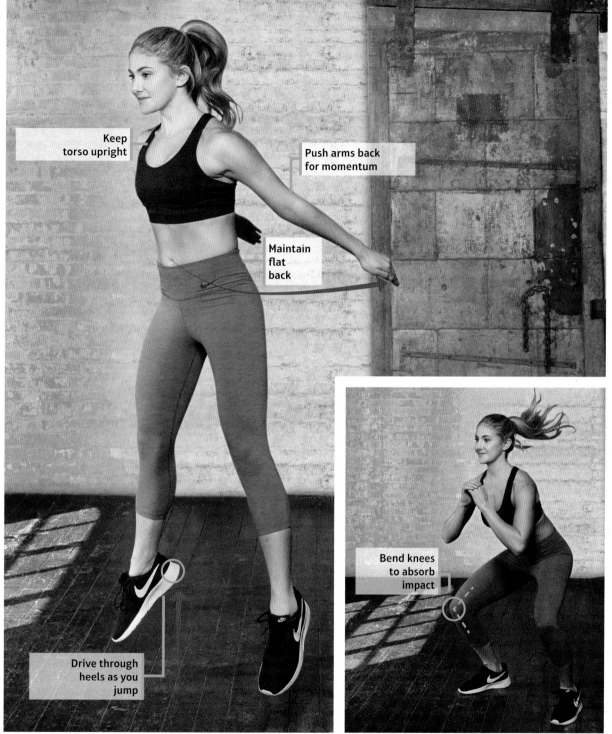

Keep torso upright

Push arms back for momentum

Maintain flat back

Drive through heels as you jump

Bend knees to absorb impact

2 Exhale, push through your heels, and straighten your legs to jump fully off the floor. Swing your arms back for momentum.

3 Swing your arms forwards and land with your feet shoulder-width apart and your toes turned out. That is one rep. Immediately transition into the next squat and repeat for the number of reps given in your workout.

BARBELL PUSH PRESS

This compound movement activates the entire body while targeting your shoulders and arms. Because you use your legs to help you push, you are able to press more weight than you would in an overhead military press.

EXERCISE PROFILE

Equipment
BARBELL

Primary muscle groups
SHOULDERS, BACK

Secondary muscle groups
CORE, TRICEPS

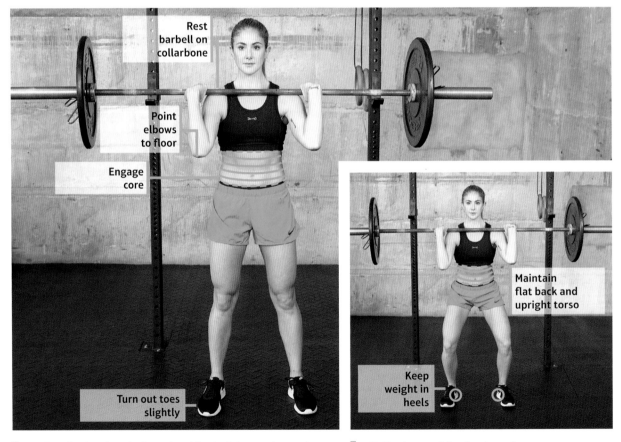

Rest barbell on collarbone

Point elbows to floor

Engage core

Turn out toes slightly

Maintain flat back and upright torso

Keep weight in heels

1 Set the bar just below shoulder height on the rack. Grasp the bar with your hands slightly wider than shoulder-width apart, palms facing up. Straighten your legs and step forwards to unrack the bar. Place your feet shoulder-width apart. Rest the bar on your collarbone.

2 Push your hips back and bend your knees to enter into a slight squat. Keep your core engaged. Inhale.

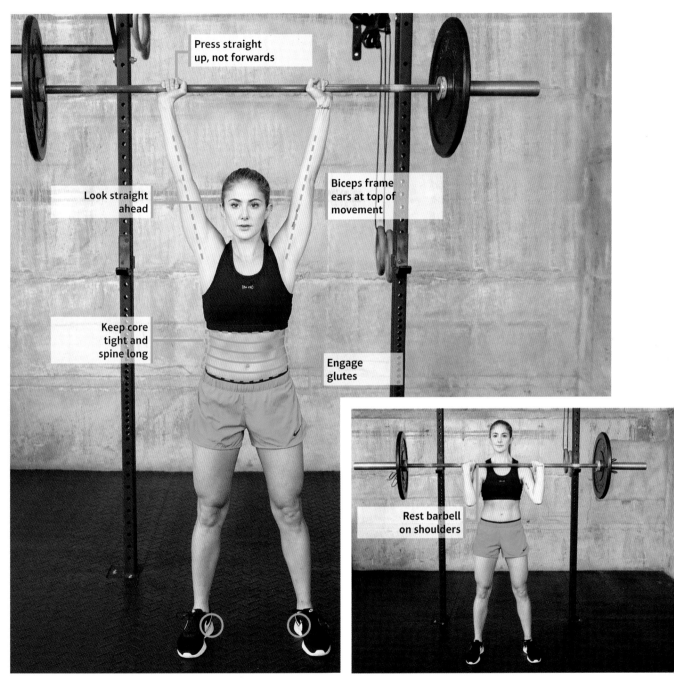

Press straight up, not forwards

Look straight ahead

Biceps frame ears at top of movement

Keep core tight and spine long

Engage glutes

Rest barbell on shoulders

3 In one swift movement, exhale, vigorously press through your heels, straighten your legs to stand up, and straighten your arms to press the barbell overhead. Keep your knees soft.

4 In a slow, controlled manner, lower the weight back to your shoulders. That is one rep. Repeat for the number of reps given in your workout.

SINGLE-ARM DUMBBELL SNATCH

In this exercise, you pull the dumbbell off the ground and press it overhead. The advanced, compound movement improves your total-body coordination and mobility. Make sure the weight is heavy enough for you to feel resistance.

EXERCISE PROFILE

Equipment
DUMBBELL

Primary muscle groups
GLUTES, HIPS, SHOULDERS

Secondary muscle groups
THIGHS, BACK, CORE

CAUTION
Do not overextend your elbow joint.

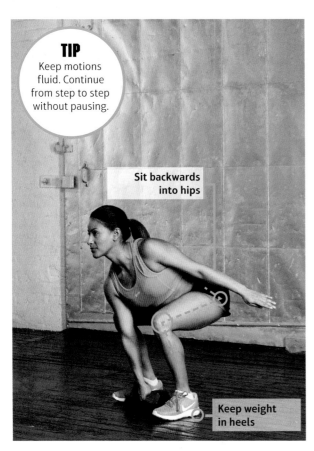

TIP
Keep motions fluid. Continue from step to step without pausing.

Sit backwards into hips

Keep weight in heels

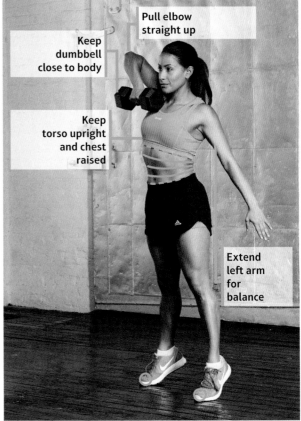

Pull elbow straight up

Keep dumbbell close to body

Keep torso upright and chest raised

Extend left arm for balance

1 Stand with your feet slightly wider than shoulder-width apart. Push your hips back and bend your knees until your thighs are parallel to the floor. Hold a dumbbell between your ankles in your right hand with an overhand grip.

2 Quickly and forcefully push your hips forwards and stand up, rising onto the balls of your feet, and pull the dumbbell straight up to your chest, guided by your elbow. Brace your core.

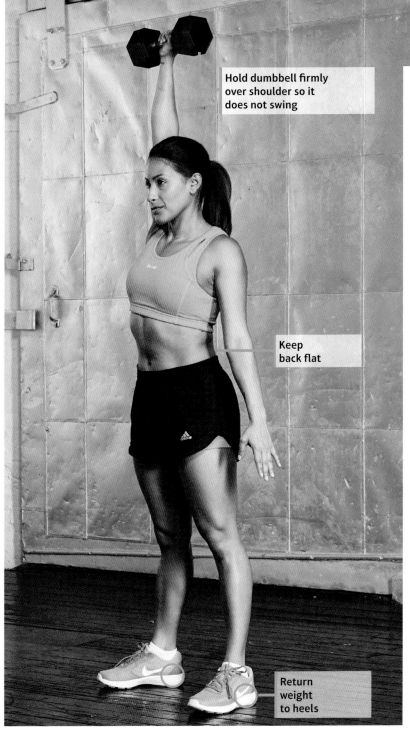

Hold dumbbell firmly over shoulder so it does not swing

Keep back flat

Return weight to heels

3 As the dumbbell reaches your shoulder, use the momentum from step 2 to extend your arm and punch the dumbbell straight up. Let your heels return to the floor.

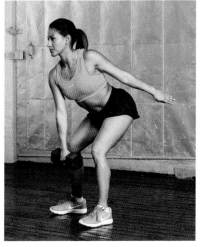

4 Carefully lower the dumbbell and return to the starting position. That is one rep.

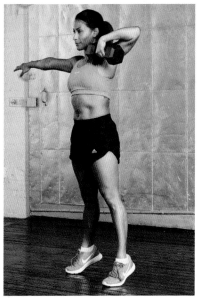

5 Perform the exercise with your left arm. That is another rep. Continue repeating the exercise, either alternating or staying on the same side for the number of reps given, according to your workout.

SINGLE-ARM KETTLEBELL CLEAN

This exercise brings the kettlebell to the racked position (resting on your collarbone), which is the first step for many kettlebell exercises. The clean tones your glutes while developing total-body strength and hip power.

EXERCISE PROFILE

Equipment
KETTLEBELL

Primary muscle groups
GLUTES, HAMSTRINGS, HIPS

Secondary muscle groups
SHOULDERS, CORE, BACK

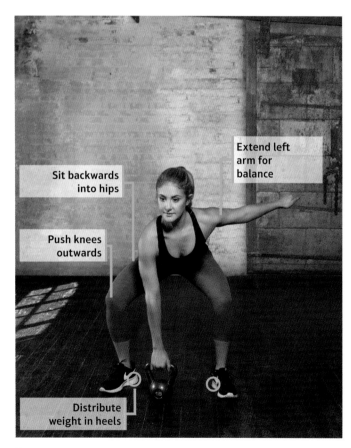

Sit backwards into hips

Extend left arm for balance

Push knees outwards

Distribute weight in heels

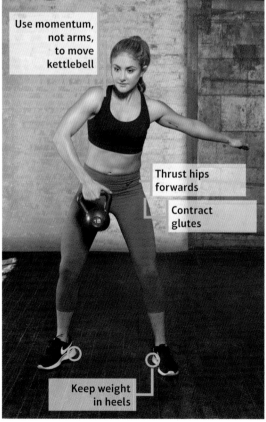

Use momentum, not arms, to move kettlebell

Thrust hips forwards

Contract glutes

Keep weight in heels

1 Stand with your feet slightly wider than shoulder-width apart. Push your hips back and bend your knees until your thighs are parallel to the floor. Hold the handle of a kettlebell between your ankles in your right hand with an overhand grip.

2 Quickly and forcefully push your hips forwards and straighten your legs. Using the momentum, guide the weight up towards your right shoulder, keeping it close to your body.

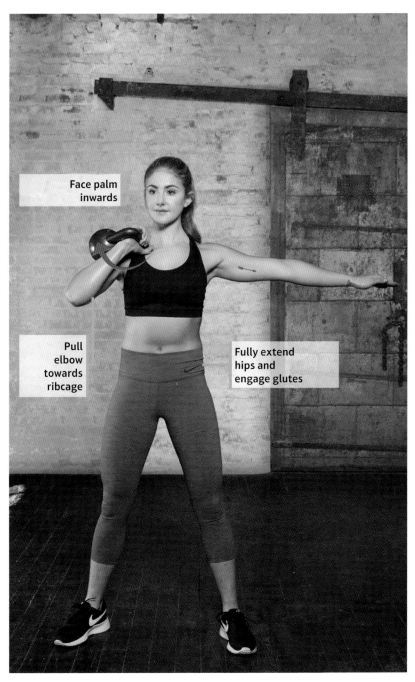

Face palm
inwards

Pull
elbow
towards
ribcage

Fully extend
hips and
engage glutes

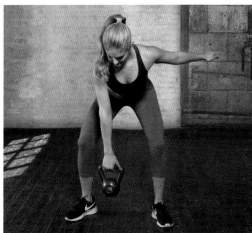

4 Carefully lower the kettlebell and return to the starting position. That is one rep.

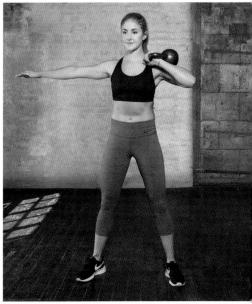

3 Pull the kettlebell up to your right shoulder, letting the kettlebell rotate around your right hand along the way. Finish with the kettlebell resting on your forearm and collarbone and your elbow close to your ribcage.

5 Perform the exercise with your left arm. That is another rep. Continue repeating the exercise, either alternating or staying on the same side for the number of reps given, according to your workout.

BARBELL CLEAN

If you aspire to strength and athleticism, this Olympic exercise will become a staple in your programme. The complex, compound movement trains you to use your entire body as a connected unit to develop power. Don't hesitate as you perform it – be powerful, fast, and fluid.

EXERCISE PROFILE

Equipment
BARBELL

Primary muscle groups
HAMSTRINGS, QUADS, SHOULDERS

Secondary muscle groups
FOREARMS, CALVES, CORE, TRICEPS

1 Place your feet under the bar, shoulder-width apart, with the bar grazing your shins. Grip the barbell so your forearms touch the outsides of your thighs. Push your glutes back and hinge forwards at the hips. Align your shoulders over the bar.

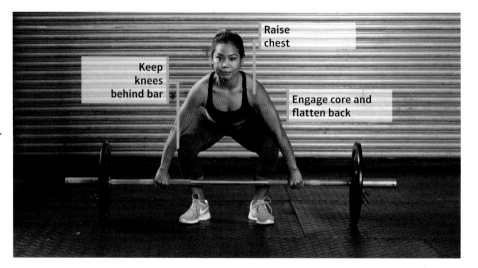

Raise chest

Keep knees behind bar

Engage core and flatten back

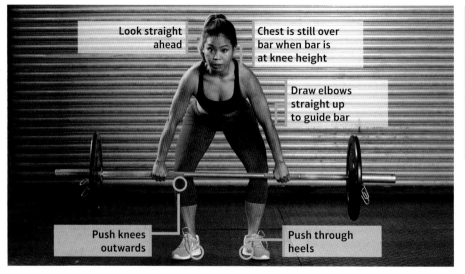

Look straight ahead

Chest is still over bar when bar is at knee height

Draw elbows straight up to guide bar

Push knees outwards

Push through heels

2 Retract your shoulder blades to activate your back, and brace your core. Inhale, push through your heels, and straighten your legs to begin to stand up. Keep the bar close to your legs.

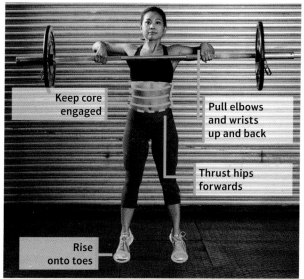

Keep core engaged

Pull elbows and wrists up and back

Thrust hips forwards

Rise onto toes

Rest barbell on collarbone

Stabilize and guide bar with arms

Use hips to squat beneath bar

Redistribute weight in heels

3 Continue standing up. When the bar passes your knees, aggressively extend your hips, legs, and ankles, and rise onto the balls of your feet. Drive the bar up to your underarms, shrug your shoulders towards your ears, and pull your elbows up and back.

4 Quickly squat down to drop your shoulders under the bar, rotate your hands and elbows underneath the bar, and catch the bar on your collarbone.

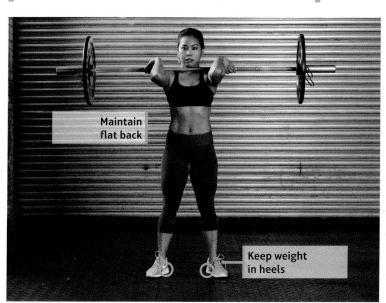

Maintain flat back

Keep weight in heels

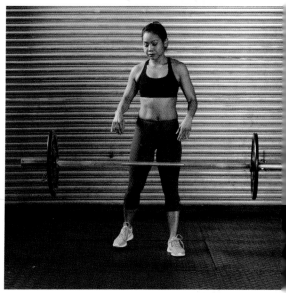

5 Immediately push through your heels to stand up with the bar on your shoulders.

6 Drop the bar to the floor. That is one rep. Repeat for the number of reps given in your workout.

RUSSIAN KETTLEBELL SWING

Swinging a heavy weight between your legs is a great way to develop hip power and glute strength. Practising this explosive hip movement helps you in nearly all other exercises and is a fast way to build athleticism.

EXERCISE PROFILE

Equipment
KETTLEBELL

Primary muscle groups
GLUTES, HAMSTRINGS, HIPS, SHOULDERS

Secondary muscle groups
CORE, BACK

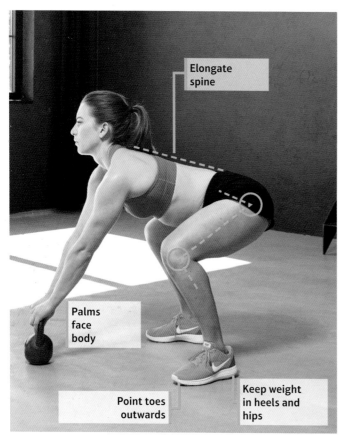

Elongate spine

Palms face body

Point toes outwards

Keep weight in heels and hips

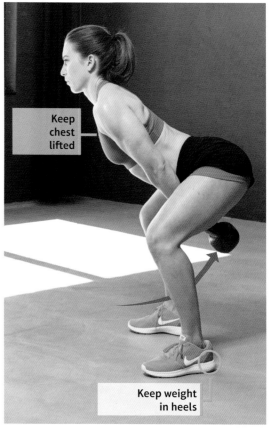

Keep chest lifted

Keep weight in heels

1 Stand with your feet wider than shoulder-width apart, and turn your toes outwards slightly. Place a kettlebell about 50cm (1¹/₂ft) in front of you. Hinge forwards at the hips, bend your knees, and grab the handle of the kettlebell with both hands.

2 Straighten your knees slightly and swing the kettlebell back between your legs.

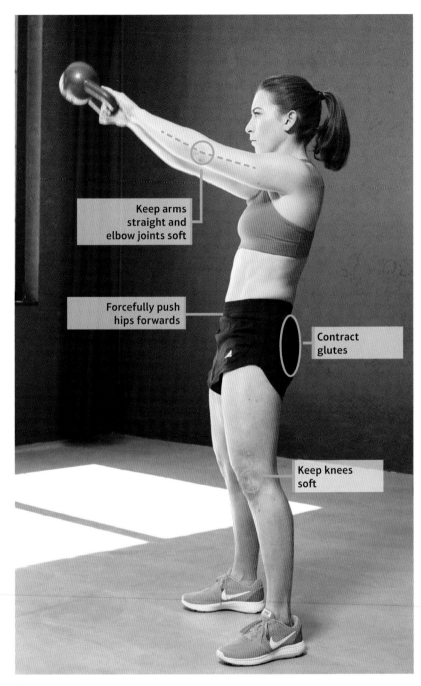

Keep arms straight and elbow joints soft

Forcefully push hips forwards

Contract glutes

Keep knees soft

3 Aggressively extend your legs and thrust your hips forwards to swing the kettlebell up to eye level. Use your glutes and hips, not your arms, to drive the movement. That is one rep.

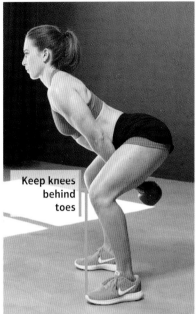

Keep knees behind toes

4 Immediately hinge forwards and push your hips back to enter into the next rep. Repeat for the number of reps given in your workout.

HARDER VARIATION

Single-arm Russian kettlebell swing
Perform the exercise as described, but use one arm at a time. Start with a lighter weight. You can switch the kettlebell quickly from hand to hand between reps, as if it is floating.

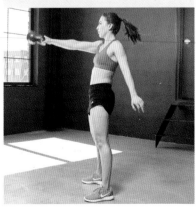

KETTLEBELL WINDMILL

Holding the kettlebell overhead while moving your torso recruits your core and hips to stabilize the weight. The kettlebell windmill is a great exercise to improve stability, mobility, and strength within the entire body.

EXERCISE PROFILE

Equipment
KETTLEBELL

Primary muscle groups
SHOULDERS, GLUTES, CORE

Secondary muscle groups
HAMSTRINGS, HIPS

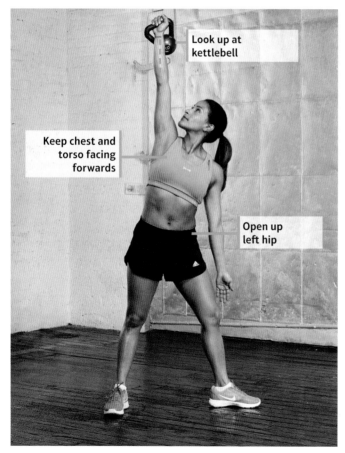

Look up at kettlebell

Keep chest and torso facing forwards

Open up left hip

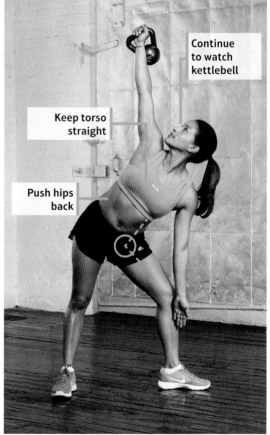

Continue to watch kettlebell

Keep torso straight

Push hips back

1 Stand with your feet wider than shoulder-width apart. Point your left foot and knee to the side. Keep your right leg facing forwards. Hold the handle of a kettlebell in your right hand, and press it straight up.

2 Begin to hinge forwards over your left leg, and push your hips back. Lean forwards, and let your left arm hang over your left foot. Keep your right arm extended in place.

TIP
This is a hip hinge, not core rotation, so do not bend or collapse torso.

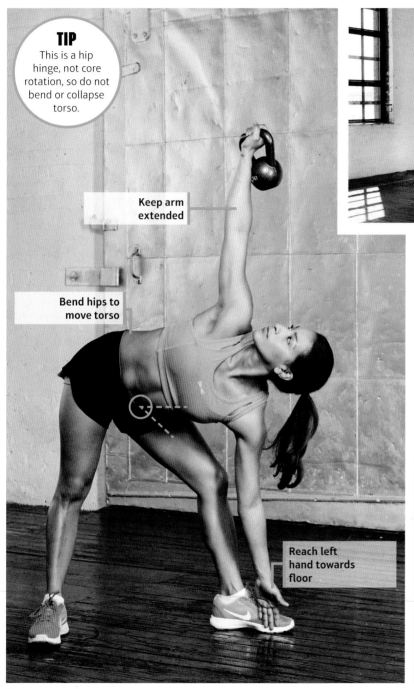

Keep arm extended

Bend hips to move torso

Reach left hand towards floor

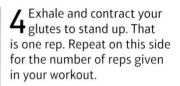

4 Exhale and contract your glutes to stand up. That is one rep. Repeat on this side for the number of reps given in your workout.

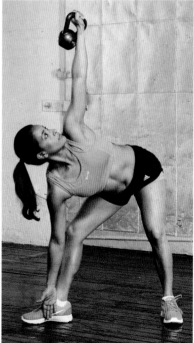

3 Continue to hinge forwards over your left leg until your torso is parallel to the floor. Feel a stretch in your left glutes. Inhale.

5 Perform the exercise on the opposite side. Repeat on this side for the number of reps given in your workout.

WALL BALL

Thrusting a heavy ball against the wall is a challenging, energy-intensive drill that tests your throwing skills and accuracy, which are often under-trained. If you squat deeply and throw with all your strength, the exercise will have your entire body exhausted and burning while improving your mobility from toes to fingertips.

EXERCISE PROFILE

Equipment
MEDICINE BALL

Primary muscle groups
LEGS, GLUTES, ARMS

Secondary muscle group
CORE

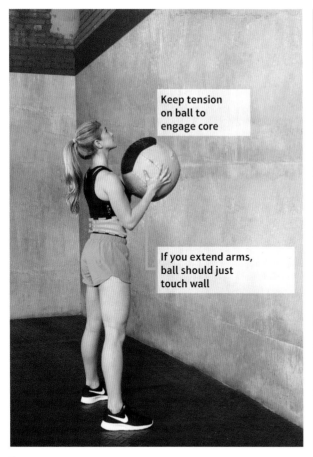

Keep tension on ball to engage core

If you extend arms, ball should just touch wall

1 Stand facing a wall with your feet wider than shoulder-width apart, and turn out your toes slightly. Hold a medicine ball at your chest.

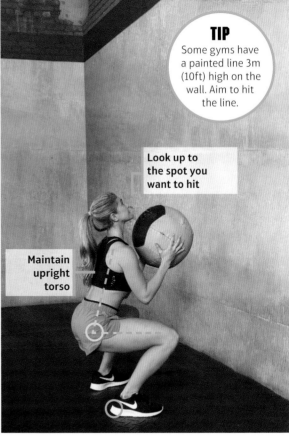

TIP
Some gyms have a painted line 3m (10ft) high on the wall. Aim to hit the line.

Look up to the spot you want to hit

Maintain upright torso

2 Push your hips back and bend your knees until your thighs are parallel to the floor. Keep your weight in your heels and hips.

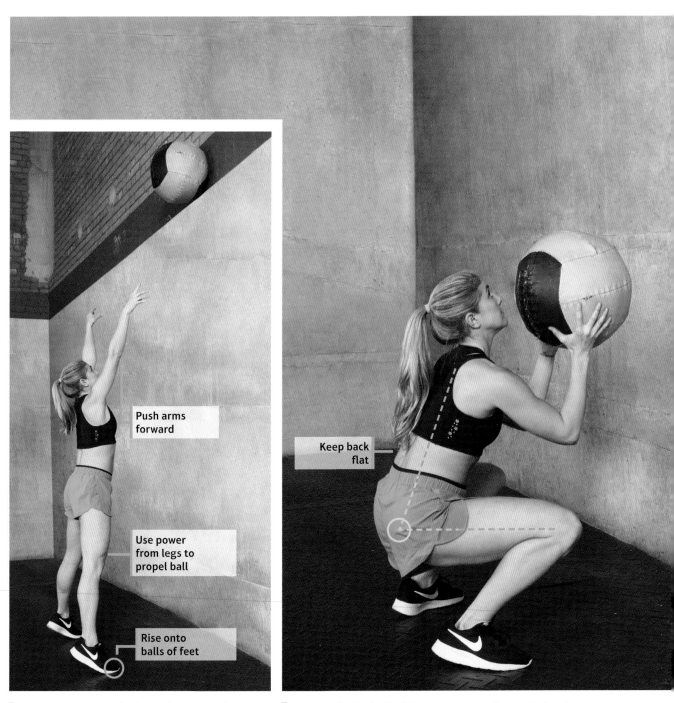

Push arms
forward

Use power
from legs to
propel ball

Rise onto
balls of feet

Keep back
flat

3 Vigorously push through your heels, stand up, and throw the ball about 3m (10ft) high against the wall. Follow through with your hands overhead.

4 Catch the ball with your extended arms. Bring it back to your chest. Immediately enter into the next rep. Repeat for the time given in your workout without letting the ball fall below your chest.

STANDING OVERHEAD
MEDICINE BALL SLAM

Forcefully throwing a medicine ball to the ground is a great way to develop power and release aggression. This exercise improves your shoulder mobility and strength while toning your abdominals and strengthening your back.

EXERCISE PROFILE

Equipment
MEDICINE BALL

Primary muscle groups
UPPER BACK, SHOULDERS

Secondary muscle groups
CORE, ARMS

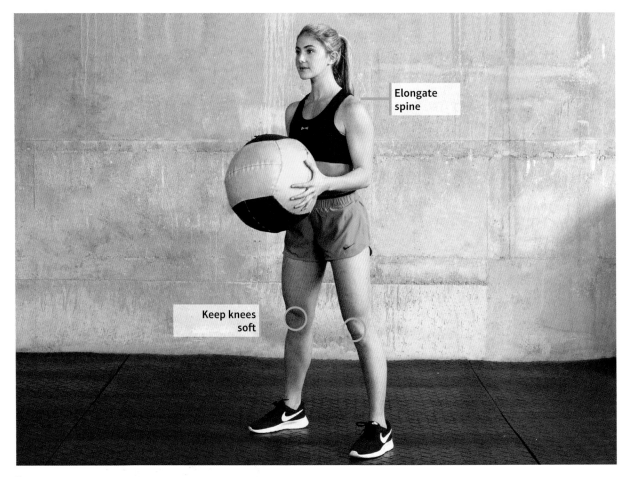

Elongate spine

Keep knees soft

1 Stand with your feet wider than shoulder-width apart, and turn out your toes slightly. Hold a medicine ball at your abdomen.

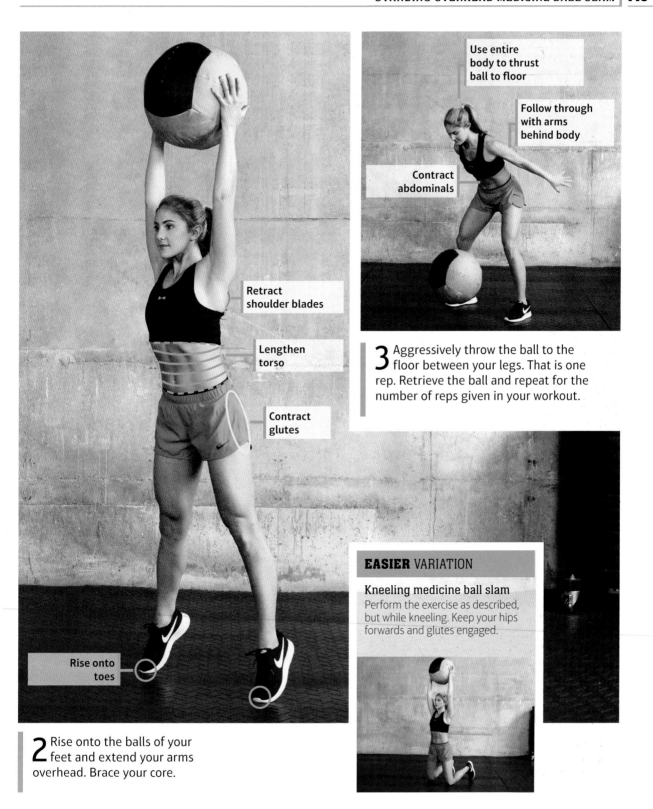

Use entire
body to thrust
ball to floor

Follow through
with arms
behind body

Contract
abdominals

Retract
shoulder blades

Lengthen
torso

Contract
glutes

3 Aggressively throw the ball to the
floor between your legs. That is one
rep. Retrieve the ball and repeat for the
number of reps given in your workout.

EASIER VARIATION

Kneeling medicine ball slam
Perform the exercise as described,
but while kneeling. Keep your hips
forwards and glutes engaged.

Rise onto
toes

2 Rise onto the balls of your
feet and extend your arms
overhead. Brace your core.

DUMBBELL THRUSTER

This is a challenging, multi-joint exercise that targets your entire body. Using free weights instead of a barbell – though it means you'll have to use less resistance – allows for a greater range of motion.

Equipment
DUMBBELLS

Primary muscle groups
QUADS, HAMSTRINGS, GLUTES, SHOULDERS, BACK

Secondary muscle group
CORE

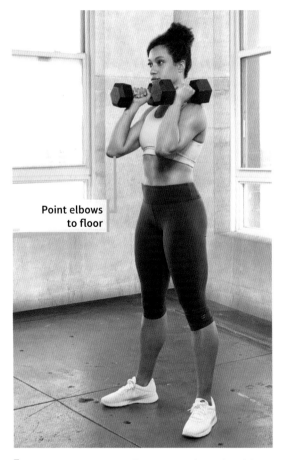

Point elbows to floor

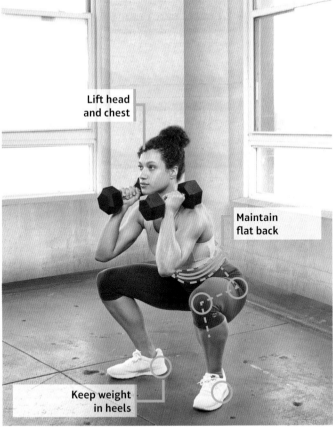

Lift head and chest

Maintain flat back

Keep weight in heels

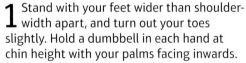

1 Stand with your feet wider than shoulder-width apart, and turn out your toes slightly. Hold a dumbbell in each hand at chin height with your palms facing inwards.

2 Inhale, brace your core, push your hips back, and bend your knees until your thighs are parallel to the floor. Keep your glutes and core engaged.

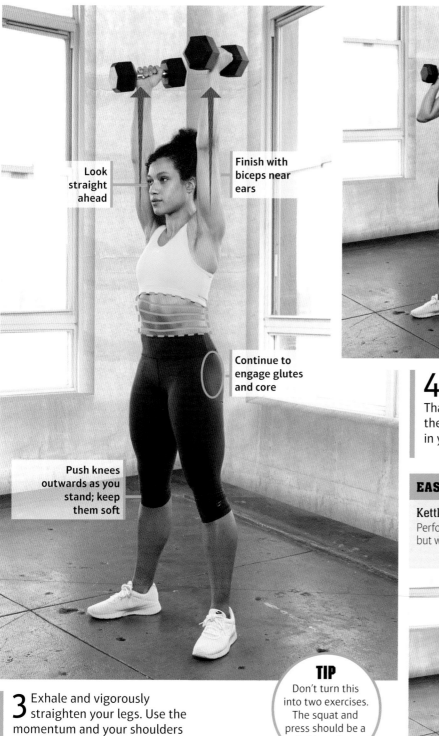

Look straight ahead

Finish with biceps near ears

Continue to engage glutes and core

Push knees outwards as you stand; keep them soft

3 Exhale and vigorously straighten your legs. Use the momentum and your shoulders to press the dumbbells overhead.

Control descent with shoulders

4 Lower the dumbbells to the starting position. That is one rep. Repeat for the number of reps given in your workout.

EASIER VARIATION

Kettlebell thruster
Perform the exercise as described, but with one kettlebell.

TIP
Don't turn this into two exercises. The squat and press should be a fluid motion.

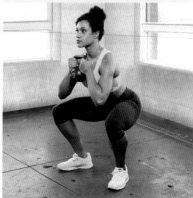

BARBELL THRUSTER

This is a great exercise for combining lower- and upper-body strength for better power and coordination. The movement is a front squat to an overhead press, which requires you to transfer power from the ground up. Keep the motions fluid.

EXERCISE PROFILE

Equipment
BARBELL

Primary muscle groups
QUADS, HAMSTRINGS, GLUTES, SHOULDERS, BACK

Secondary muscle group
CORE

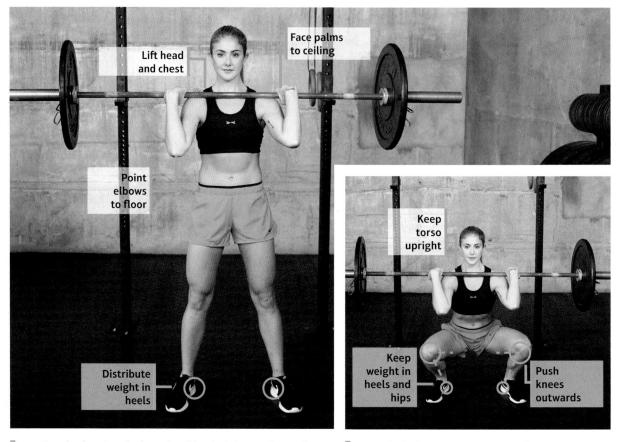

Lift head and chest

Face palms to ceiling

Point elbows to floor

Distribute weight in heels

Keep torso upright

Keep weight in heels and hips

Push knees outwards

1 Set the bar just below shoulder height on the rack. Grasp the bar with your hands slightly wider than shoulder-width apart, palms facing up. Straighten your legs and step forwards to unrack the bar. Place your feet shoulder-width apart. Rest the bar on your collarbone.

2 Inhale, brace your core, push your hips back, and bend your knees until your thighs are parallel to the floor.

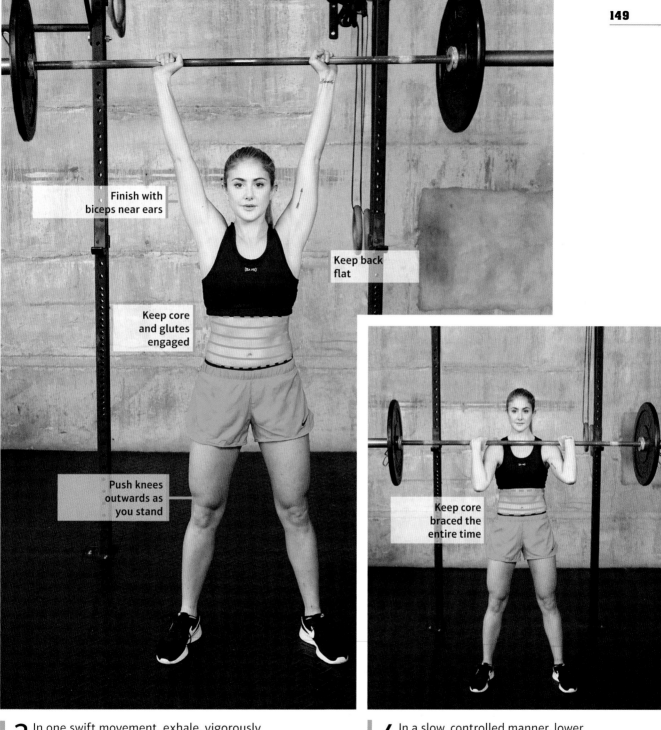

Finish with biceps near ears

Keep back flat

Keep core and glutes engaged

Push knees outwards as you stand

Keep core braced the entire time

3 In one swift movement, exhale, vigorously push your hips forwards, and straighten your legs. Use the momentum and your shoulders to press the barbell overhead.

4 In a slow, controlled manner, lower the bar back to your shoulders. That is one rep. Repeat for the number of reps given in your workout.

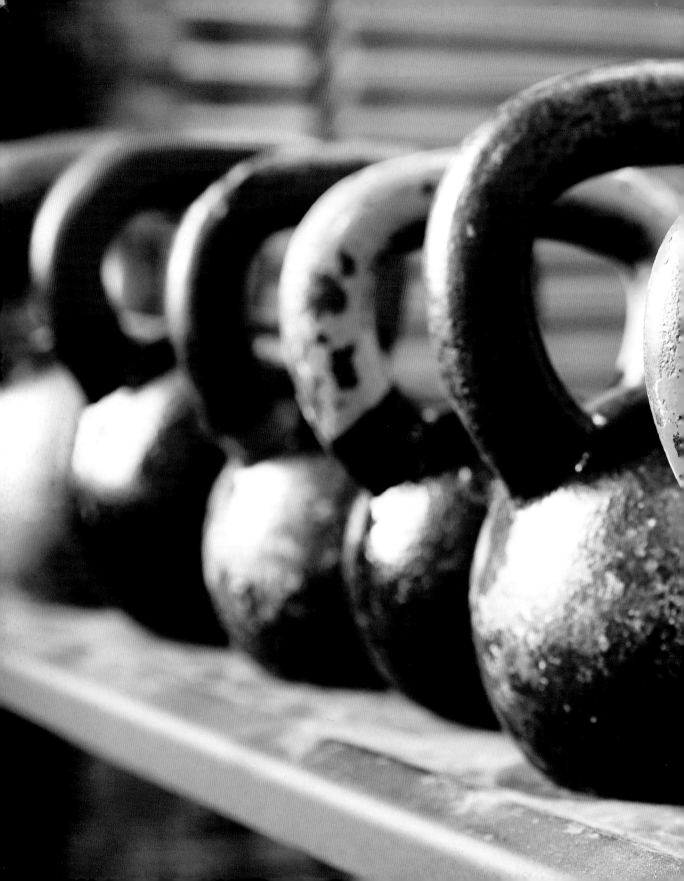

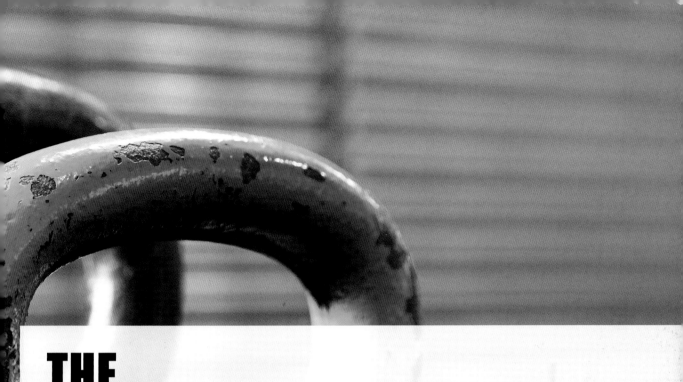
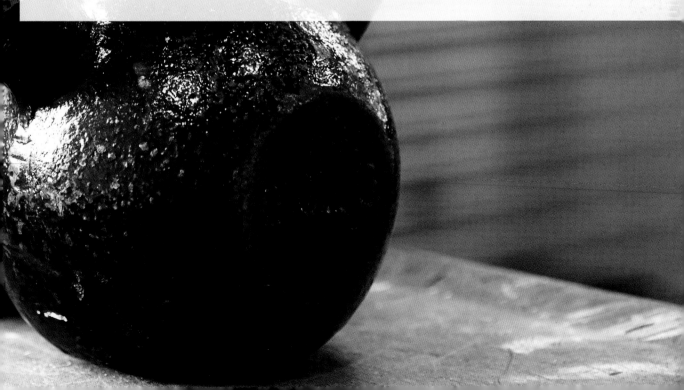

THE
PROGRAMMES

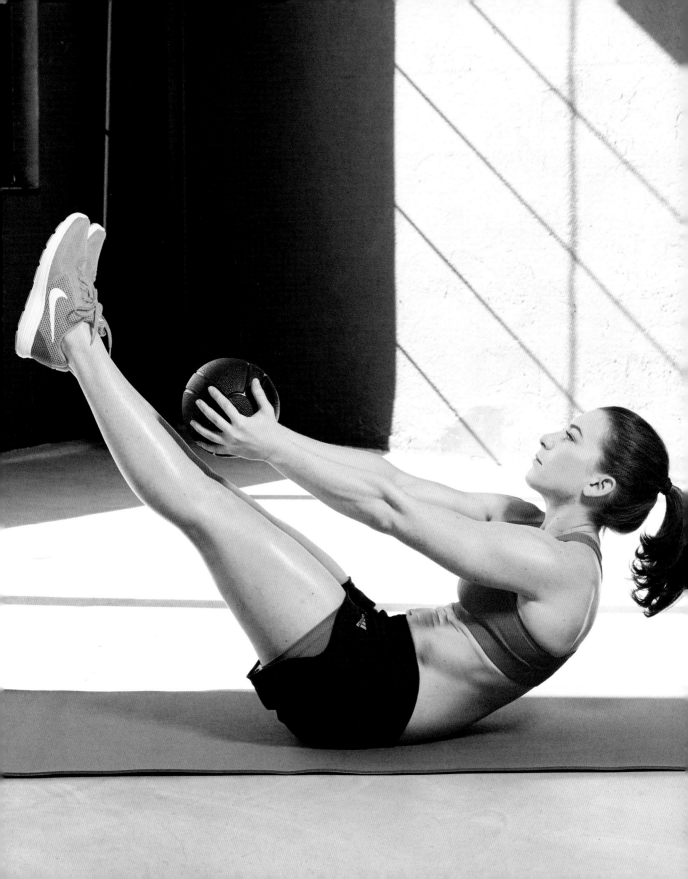

LEVEL 1 Weeks 1–4

Start your 12-week programme with this 4-week foundation phase, which prepares your muscles for heavier weights and more intense training to come. Follow the weekly schedule, repeating it for a total of 4 consecutive weeks. The workouts are on the following pages. Don't forget to also perform the warm-up and cool-down sequences (pp26–29) on every workout day. After completing all 4 weeks, advance to Level 1: Weeks 5–8.

WEEKLY SCHEDULE

DAY 1	Upper body – push
DAY 2	Lower body – deadlift
DAY 3	Rest
DAY 4	Upper body – pull
DAY 5	Lower body – squat
DAY 6	Rest
DAY 7	Cardio

Rest days
You have 2 days to rest during each week of this phase. You can move them around within each week to accommodate your schedule. Push yourself during the workouts so these rest days feel worth it. A rest day is not an inactive day; it's simply a rest day from weights and intense cardio. Take a yoga class or go for a walk, and keep your body moving!

Cardio day
Your cardio day should be in the form of HIIT, which will blast calories in a short period of time. With a rower or treadmill, alternate between intervals of high-intensity work (sprinting) and low-intensity rest (jogging or walking). Start with a ratio of 30 seconds' work to 90 seconds' rest, and gradually advance to 30 seconds' work to 60 seconds' rest.

DAY 1 Upper body – push

Begin the week by challenging your entire upper body, focusing on pushing movements with your arms. Each circuit includes a core exercise to fire up your abdominals.

SUPERSET

Perform the exercises back to back for the specified number of reps. Rest and repeat as indicated.		
Push-up	**8** reps	p82
Bodyweight Russian twist	**16** reps	p55
Rest for 60 seconds		
Repeat twice for a total of 3 sets		

CIRCUIT 1

For each circuit, perform the exercises back to back for the specified number of reps. Rest and repeat as indicated.		
Standing dumbbell shoulder press	**8** reps	p74
Triceps dip	**8** reps	p86
Butterfly sit-up	**10** reps	p38
Rest for 60 seconds		
Repeat twice for a total of 3 rounds		

CIRCUIT 2

Standing dual-dumbbell biceps curl	**10** reps	p88
Lying dumbbell chest fly	**10** reps	p76
High plank shoulder tap (alternating)	**16** reps	p46
Rest for 60 seconds		
Repeat twice for a total of 3 rounds		

DAY 2 Lower body – deadlift

Your legs and hips are the foundation for most movements. This workout begins with a basic hinge-pattern movement – the deadlift – then adds metabolic exercises to challenge your heart.

MAIN LIFT

Complete 2 warm-up sets with a light kettlebell. Then do 3 working sets with a challenging kettlebell (the last 2 reps should be very difficult).		
Kettlebell deadlift (light)	**5** reps	p113
Rest for 60 seconds		
Repeat once for a total of 2 warm-up sets		
Kettlebell deadlift (heavy)	**8** reps	p113
Rest for 90 seconds		
Repeat twice for a total of 3 working sets		

CIRCUIT 1

For each circuit, perform the exercises back to back for the specified number of reps or secs. Rest and repeat as indicated.		
Bodyweight squat	**10** reps	p93
Dumbbell step-up (without alternating)	**8** reps/leg	p110
Fast mountain climber	**30** secs	p56
Rest for 60 seconds		
Repeat twice for a total of 3 rounds		

CIRCUIT 2

Kettlebell single-leg deadlift (without alternating)	**8** reps/leg	p116
Bodyweight reverse lunge (alternating)	**16** reps	p107
Jump squat	**8** reps	p128
Rest for 60 seconds		
Repeat twice for a total of 3 rounds		

DAY 3

Rest

DAY 4 Upper body – pull

A strong back is a huge source of power and ensures good posture and healthy movement. This workout focuses on the back muscles, along with core exercises to challenge the whole body.

SUPERSET

Perform the exercises back to back for the specified number of reps. Rest and repeat as indicated.		
Ring row	**8** reps	p69
Kneeling medicine ball slam	**10** reps	p145
Rest for 60 seconds		
Repeat twice for a total of 3 sets		

CIRCUIT

Perform the exercises back to back for the specified number of reps. Rest and repeat as indicated.		
Staggered stance single-arm row (without alternating)	**8** reps/arm	p62
Dumbbell upright row	**10** reps	p68
Bodyweight toe touch	**12** reps	p35
Rest for 60 seconds		
Repeat twice for a total of 3 rounds		

CORE FINISHER

Perform the exercises back to back for the specified number of reps. Rest and repeat as indicated.		
Kettlebell plank drag	**10** reps	p48
Side plank hip drop (without alternating)	**8** reps/side	p50
Bicycle crunch	**16** reps	p32
Rest for 45 seconds		
Repeat 3 times for a total of 4 rounds		

DAY 5 Lower body – squat

This is the hardest workout of the week, but don't worry – you get to rest tomorrow. The lower-body work will set your legs on fire, and the core finisher will leave you exhausted.

SUPERSET

Perform the exercises back to back, pushing yourself to hold the plank for as long as you're able. Rest and repeat as indicated.		
Kettlebell goblet squat	**8** reps	p96
Forearm plank hold	As long as you can	p45
Rest for 60 seconds		
Repeat twice for a total of 3 sets		

CIRCUIT

Perform the exercises back to back for the specified number of reps. Rest and repeat as indicated.		
Dumbbell Romanian deadlift	**10** reps	p114
Bodyweight reverse lunge (alternating)	**16** reps	p107
Jump lunge	**20** reps	p124
Rest for 60 seconds		
Repeat twice for a total of 3 rounds		

CORE FINISHER

Perform the exercises back to back for the specified number of reps. Rest and repeat as indicated.		
Slow cross mountain climber (alternating)	**16** reps	p58
V-up	**8** reps	p36
Bicycle crunch	**16** reps	p32
Forearm plank leg march (alternating)	**16** reps	p44
Rest for 45 seconds		
Repeat twice for a total of 3 rounds		

DAY 6

Rest

DAY 7

Cardio

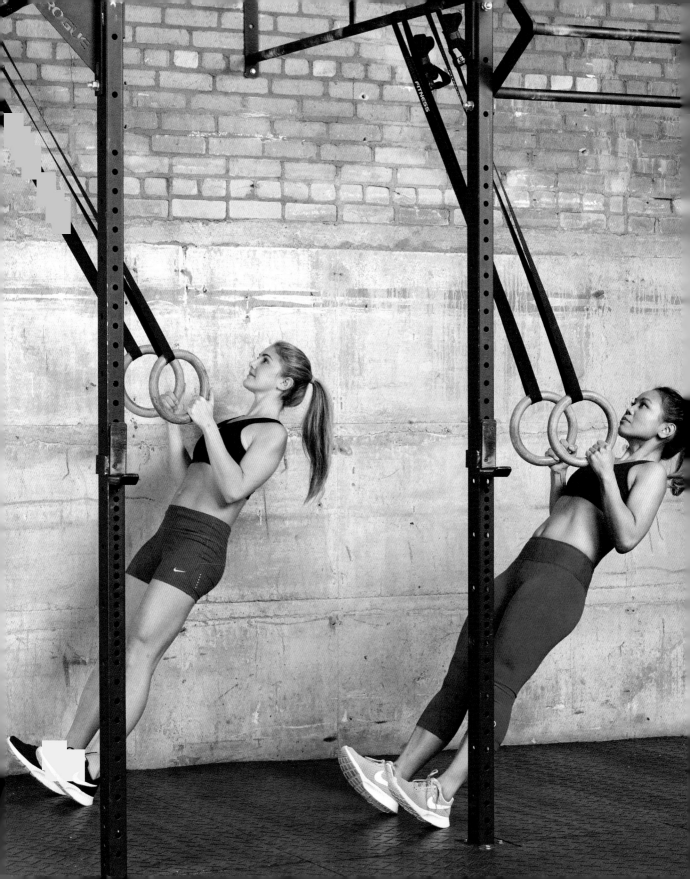

LEVEL 1 Weeks 5-8

The intensity builds during these weeks with more timed exercises. Push yourself to complete more reps than you did during the last phase. Follow the weekly schedule, repeating it for a total of 4 consecutive weeks. The workouts are on the following pages. Don't forget to also perform the warm-up and cool-down sequences (pp26-29) on every workout day. After completing all 4 weeks, advance to Level 1: Weeks 9-12.

WEEKLY SCHEDULE

DAY 1	Upper body – push
DAY 2	Lower body – single-leg focus
DAY 3	Rest
DAY 4	Upper body – pull
DAY 5	Lower body – deadlift
DAY 6	Rest
DAY 7	Cardio

Rest days
You again have 2 days to rest during each week of this phase. You can move them around within each week to accommodate your schedule. Push yourself during the workouts so these rest days feel worth it. A rest day is not an inactive day; it's simply a rest day from weights and intense cardio. Take a yoga class or go for a walk, and keep your body moving!

Cardio day
Your cardio day should be in the form of HIIT, which will blast calories in a short period of time. With a rower or treadmill, alternate between intervals of high-intensity work (sprinting) and low-intensity rest (jogging or walking). Start with a ratio of 30 seconds' work to 60 seconds' rest, and gradually advance to 30 seconds' work to 30 seconds' rest. You can also add incline or bodyweight movements to your rest intervals. For example, after every 5 minutes on the machine, hold a 30-second plank or perform 10 bodyweight squats.

DAY 1 Upper body – push

From push-ups to front squats, healthy shoulders are the foundation for upper-body fitness. Use this workout to target your shoulders and chest while challenging your entire upper body.

SUPERSET 1

For each superset, perform the exercises back to back for the specified number of reps or secs. Rest and repeat as indicated.		
Dual-kettlebell push press	**8** reps	p126
V-up	**30** secs	p36
Rest for 45 seconds		
Repeat twice for a total of 3 sets		

SUPERSET 2

Dumbbell upright row	**10** reps	p68
Standing dumbbell Arnold press	**10** reps	p75
Rest for 60 seconds		
Repeat twice for a total of 3 sets		

CIRCUIT 1

For each circuit, perform the exercises back to back for the specified number of reps or secs. Rest and repeat as indicated.		
T push-up (alternating)	**30** secs	p84
Triceps dip	**12** reps	p86
High plank shoulder tap (alternating)	**20** reps	p46
Rest for 60 seconds		
Repeat twice for a total of 3 rounds		

CIRCUIT 2

Lying dumbbell chest fly	**10** reps	p76
Single-arm half-kneeling kettlebell press (without alternating)	**10** reps/ arm	p72
Side plank warm hug (without alternating)	**10** reps/ arm	p52
Rest for 60 seconds		
Repeat twice for a total of 3 rounds		

DAY 2 Lower body – single-leg focus

Today is all about single-leg power. These exercises work one leg at a time to sharpen your central nervous system and improve your balance and stability.

SUPERSET

Perform the exercises back to back for the specified number of reps or secs. Rest and repeat as indicated.		
Bodyweight RFE split squat (without alternating)	**8** reps/ side	p99
Butterfly sit-up	**30** secs	p38
Rest for 60 seconds		
Repeat twice for a total of 3 sets		

CIRCUIT 1

For each circuit, perform the exercises back to back for the specified number of reps or secs. Rest and repeat as indicated.		
Kettlebell single-leg deadlift (without alternating)	**8** reps/ leg	p116
Dumbbell lateral lunge (alternating)	**20** reps	p108
Jump lunge	**30** secs	p124
Rest for 60 seconds		
Repeat twice for a total of 3 rounds		

CIRCUIT 2

Dumbbell Romanian deadlift	**10** reps	p114
Kettlebell goblet squat	**10** reps	p96
Slow cross mountain climber (alternating)	**20** reps	p58
Dumbbell walking lunge	**60** secs	p104
Rest for 60 seconds		
Repeat twice for a total of 3 rounds		

DAY 3

Rest

DAY 4 Upper body – pull

This workout challenges your back, biceps, and core. To burn calories, make sure that you move quickly through the circuits, and take rests only when prescribed.

SUPERSET	Perform the exercises back to back for the specified number of reps or secs. Rest and repeat as indicated.		
	Staggered stance single-arm row (without alternating)	**8** reps/arm	p62
	Slow cross mountain climber (alternating)	**30** secs	p58
	Rest for 45 seconds		
	Repeat twice for a total of 3 sets		

CIRCUIT 1	For each circuit, perform the exercises back to back for the specified number of reps or secs. Rest and repeat as indicated.		
	Standing dual-dumbbell biceps curl	**10** reps	p88
	Dumbbell renegade row (alternating)	**16** reps	p64
	Kneeling medicine ball slam	**30** secs	p145
	Rest for 60 seconds		
	Repeat twice for a total of 3 rounds		

CIRCUIT 2	Ring row	**10** reps	p69
	Kettlebell plank drag	**10** reps	p48
	High plank shoulder tap (alternating)	**20** reps	p46
	Kettlebell farmer's walk	**20** steps	p60
	Burpee	**10** reps	p118
	Rest for 60 seconds		
	Repeat three times for a total of 4 rounds		

DAY 5 Lower body – deadlift

These lower-body focused circuits require you to push forcefully into the ground for every exercise. Imagine your power originating from the ground and travelling upwards through your body.

MAIN LIFT	Complete 2 warm-up sets with a light resistance. Then do 3 working sets with a challenging resistance (the last 2 reps should be very difficult).		
	Conventional barbell deadlift (light)	**8** reps	p112
	Rest for 60 seconds		
	Repeat once for a total of 2 warm-up sets		
	Conventional barbell deadlift (heavy)	**10** reps	p112
	Rest for 90 seconds		
	Repeat twice for a total of 3 working sets		

CIRCUIT 1	For each circuit, perform the exercises back to back for the specified number of reps. Rest and repeat as indicated.		
	Kettlebell goblet squat	**10** reps	p96
	Dumbbell step-up (without alternating)	**8** reps/leg	p110
	Forearm plank leg march (alternating)	**20** reps	p44
	Rest for 60 seconds		
	Repeat twice for a total of 3 rounds		

CIRCUIT 2	Kettlebell single-leg deadlift (without alternating)	**8** reps/leg	p116
	Dumbbell reverse lunge (alternating)	**16** reps	p106
	Box jump	**10** reps	p122
	Rest for 60 seconds		
	Repeat twice for a total of 3 rounds		

DAY 6
Rest

DAY 7
Cardio

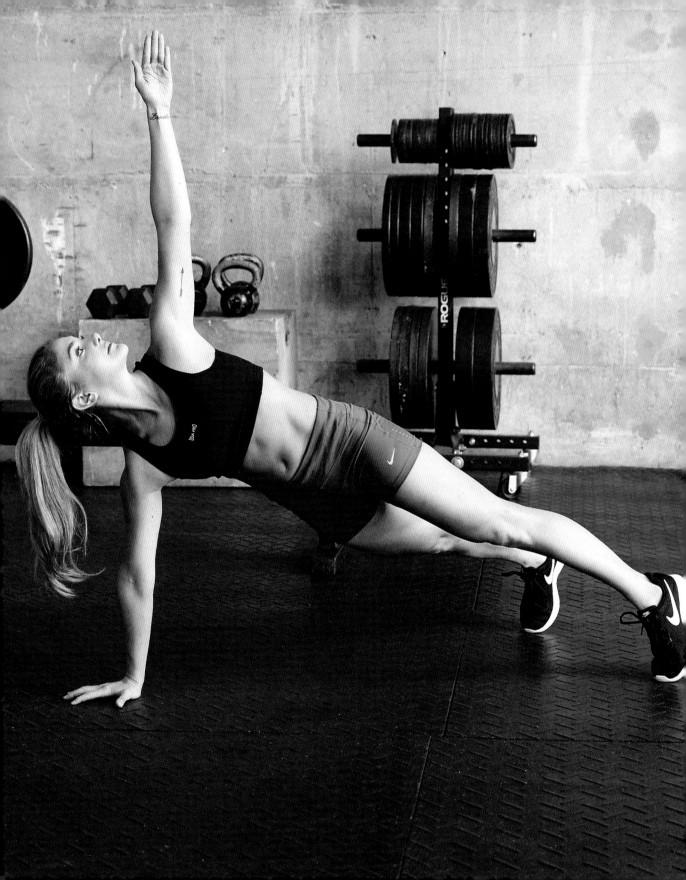

LEVEL 1 Weeks 9–12

In this final phase of Level 1, there is a cardio finisher circuit at the end of each workout. This metabolic conditioning means you'll continue burning calories long after you leave the gym. Follow the weekly schedule, repeating it for a total of 4 consecutive weeks. The workouts are on the following pages. Don't forget to also perform the warm-up and cool-down sequences (pp26–29) on every workout day. After completing all 4 weeks, reassess your fitness and either repeat Level 1 or advance to Level 2.

WEEKLY SCHEDULE

DAY 1	Upper body – push
DAY 2	Lower body – deadlift
DAY 3	Cardio
DAY 4	Upper body – pull
DAY 5	Lower body – squat
DAY 6	Rest
DAY 7	Cardio

Rest day

You have 1 day to rest during each week of this phase. You can move it around within each week to accommodate your schedule. Push yourself during the workouts so the rest day feels worth it. A rest day is not an inactive day; it's simply a rest day from weights and intense cardio. Take a yoga class or go for a walk, and keep your body moving!

Cardio days

One of your days should be in the form of HIIT, which will blast calories in a short period of time. With a rower or treadmill, alternate between intervals of high-intensity work (sprinting) and low-intensity rest (jogging or walking). Start with a ratio of 30 seconds' work to 60 seconds' rest, and gradually advance to 30 seconds' work to 30 seconds' rest. You can also add incline or bodyweight movements to your rest intervals. For example, after every 5 minutes on the machine, hold a 30-second plank or perform 10 bodyweight squats.

For the other day, use cardio equipment or go for a jog outside. Keep the intensity and pace moderate and consistent throughout.

LEVEL 1 Weeks 9–12

DAY 1 Upper body – push

Start your workout with the complex bench press, and maintain the intensity all the way through to your cardio finisher. These circuits will tone many of your upper-body pushing muscles.

MAIN LIFT

Complete 1 warm-up set with a light resistance. Then do 3 working sets with a challenging resistance (the last 2 reps should be very difficult).

Barbell bench press (light)	**6** reps	p70
Rest for 45 seconds		
Do not repeat warm-up set		
Barbell bench press (heavy)	**8–12** reps	p70
Rest for up to 2 minutes		
Repeat twice for a total of 3 working sets		

CIRCUIT 1

For each circuit, perform the exercises back to back for the specified number of reps. Rest and repeat as indicated.

Lying dumbbell chest fly	**12** reps	p76
Dual-kettlebell push press	**10** reps	p126
T push-up (alternating)	**10** reps	p84
Rest for 60 seconds		
Repeat twice for a total of 3 rounds		

CIRCUIT 2

Standing dual-dumbbell biceps curl	**8** reps	p88
Triceps dip	**12** reps	p86
High plank shoulder tap (alternating)	**20** reps	p46
Rest for 60 seconds		
Repeat twice for a total of 3 rounds		

METABOLIC FINISHER

Chipper: perform the exercises back to back for the specified number of reps, decreasing your reps by 2 each round.

Russian kettlebell swing	**10 (8, 6, 4, 2)** reps	p138
Kneeling medicine ball slam	**10 (8, 6, 4, 2)** reps	p145
Do not rest between rounds		
Repeat 4 times for a total of 5 rounds		

DAY 2 Lower body – deadlift

Today's deadlifts and squats will have your glutes and hamstrings exhausted. The pulling motions through your posterior chain will make all your movements healthier and stronger.

MAIN LIFT

Complete 2 warm-up sets with a light resistance. Then do 3 working sets with a challenging resistance (the last 2 reps should be very difficult).

Conventional barbell deadlift (light)	**5** reps	p112
Rest for 60 seconds		
Repeat once for a total of 2 warm-up sets		
Conventional barbell deadlift (heavy)	**8** reps	p112
Rest for up to 2 minutes		
Repeat twice for a total of 3 working sets		

CIRCUIT 1

For each circuit, perform the exercises back to back for the specified number of reps or secs. Rest and repeat as indicated.

Dumbbell sumo squat	**10** reps	p94
Dumbbell lateral lunge (without alternating)	**10** reps/side	p108
Fast mountain climber	**30** secs	p56
Rest for 60 seconds		
Repeat twice for a total of 3 rounds		

CIRCUIT 2

Rear-foot-elevated split squat (without alternating)	**8** reps/side	p98
Dumbbell Romanian deadlift	**10** reps	p114
Jump squat	**30** secs	p128
Rest for 60 seconds		
Repeat twice for a total of 3 rounds		

METABOLIC FINISHER

Chipper: perform the exercises back to back for the specified number of reps, decreasing your reps by 3 each round.

Box jump	**15 (12, 9)** reps	p122
Russian kettlebell swing	**15 (12, 9)** reps	p138
Do not rest between rounds		
Repeat twice for a total of 3 rounds		

DAY 3

Cardio

DAY 4 Upper body – pull

This workout targets those muscles that let you pull with your arms. It is the perfect counterpart to the work you did on Day 1 to help you build a healthy upper-body system.

MAIN LIFT

Complete 1 warm-up set with a light resistance. Then do 3 working sets with a challenging resistance (the last 2 reps should be very difficult).		
Barbell bent-over row (light)	**6** reps	p66
Rest for 45 seconds		
Do not repeat warm-up set		
Barbell bent-over row (heavy)	**8** reps	p66
Rest for up to 2 minutes		
Repeat twice for a total of 3 working sets		

CIRCUIT 1

For each circuit, perform the exercises back to back for the specified number of reps. Rest and repeat as indicated.		
Ring row	**12** reps	p69
Standing dual-dumbbell biceps curl	**12** reps	p88
Kettlebell plank drag	**10** reps	p48
Rest for 60 seconds		
Repeat twice for a total of 3 rounds		

CIRCUIT 2

Staggered stance single-arm row (without alternating)	**10** reps/arm	p62
Dual-kettlebell push press	**8** reps	p126
Dumbbell toe touch	**10** reps	p34
Rest for 60 seconds		
Repeat twice for a total of 3 rounds		

METABOLIC FINISHER

Perform the exercises back to back for the specified number of reps or secs. Rest and repeat as indicated.		
Dumbbell renegade row (alternating)	**16** reps	p64
Single-arm dumbbell snatch (alternating)	**16** reps	p132
Fast mountain climber	**30** secs	p56
Burpee	**10** reps	p118
Rest for 45 seconds		
Repeat 3 times for a total of 4 rounds		

DAY 5 Lower body – squat

Today is all about the squat. Complete these circuits to shape your lower body and develop leg strength and power. Finish with burpees to make your metabolism skyrocket.

MAIN LIFT

Complete 2 warm-up sets with a light resistance. Then do 3 working sets with a challenging resistance (the last 2 reps should be very difficult).		
Barbell front squat (light)	**5** reps	p90
Rest for 45 seconds		
Repeat once for a total of 2 warm-up sets		
Barbell front squat (heavy)	**8** reps	p90
Rest for up to 2 minutes		
Repeat twice for a total of 3 working sets		

CIRCUIT 1

For each circuit, perform the exercises back to back for the specified number of reps or steps. Rest and repeat as indicated.		
Dumbbell sumo squat	**10** reps	p94
Dumbbell walking lunge	**20** steps	p104
Side plank hip drop (without alternating)	**10** reps/side	p50
Rest for 60 seconds		
Repeat twice for a total of 3 rounds		

CIRCUIT 2

Kettlebell goblet squat	**10** reps	p96
Dumbbell lateral lunge (without alternating)	**10** reps/side	p108
Jump squat	**10** reps	p128
Rest for 60 seconds		
Repeat twice for a total of 3 rounds		

METABOLIC FINISHER

5-minute EMOM: Using a stopwatch to monitor time, perform 10 reps of the exercise every minute on the minute for 5 minutes total. Rest for the remainder of every minute.		
Burpee	**10** reps	p118
Rest until the minute mark		
Repeat for a total of 5 minutes		

DAY 6 Rest

DAY 7 Cardio

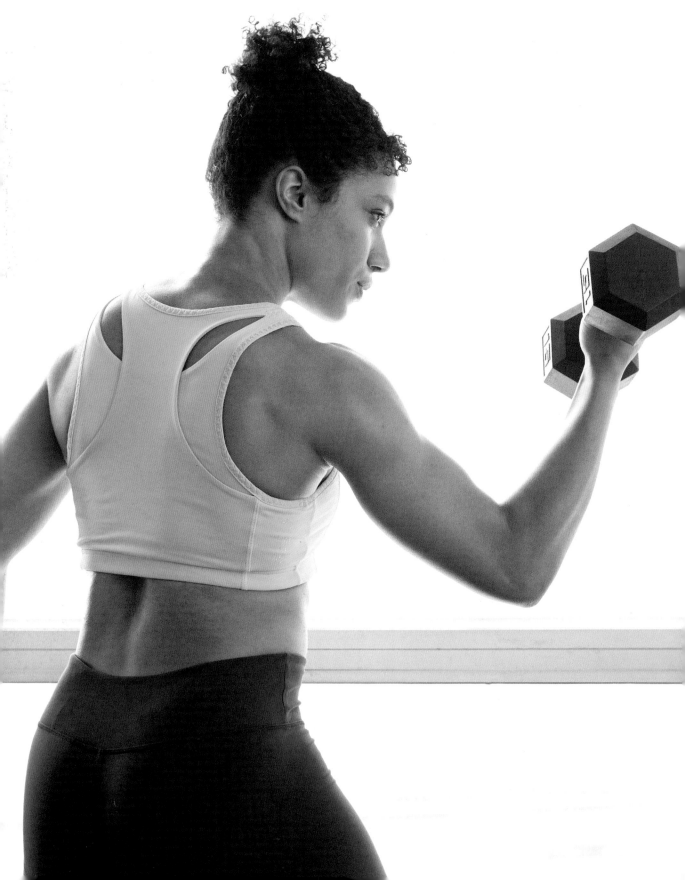

LEVEL 2 Weeks 1–4

During this first 4-week phase, the high rep counts will improve the endurance of your muscles and prepare you to use heavier resistance in the upcoming phases. Follow the weekly schedule, repeating it for a total of 4 consecutive weeks. The workouts are on the following pages. Don't forget to also perform the warm-up and cool-down sequences (pp26–29) on every workout day. After completing all 4 weeks, advance to Level 2: Weeks 5–8.

WEEKLY SCHEDULE

DAY 1	Upper body – push
DAY 2	Lower body – deadlift
DAY 3	Rest
DAY 4	Upper body – pull
DAY 5	Lower body – squat
DAY 6	Rest
DAY 7	Cardio

Rest days
You have 2 days to rest during each week of this phase. You can move them around within each week to accommodate your schedule. Push yourself during the workouts so these rest days feel worth it. A rest day is not an inactive day; it's simply a rest day from weights and intense cardio. Take a yoga class or go for a walk, and keep your body moving!

Cardio day
Your cardio day should be in the form of HIIT, which will blast calories in a short period of time. With a rower or treadmill, alternate between intervals of high-intensity work (sprinting) and low-intensity rest (jogging or walking). Start with a ratio of 30 seconds' work to 60 seconds' rest, and gradually advance to 30 seconds' work to 30 seconds' rest.

DAY 1 Upper body – push

Start off Level 2 with the bench press, which works the entire upper body at once. The following circuits will then isolate and shape the individual muscles.

MAIN LIFT

Complete 2 warm-up sets with a light resistance. Then do 3 working sets with a challenging resistance (the last 2 reps should be very difficult).

Barbell bench press (light)	**5** reps	p70
Rest for 60 seconds		
Repeat once for a total of 2 warm-up sets		
Barbell bench press (heavy)	**8–10** reps	p70
Rest for up to 2 minutes		
Repeat twice for a total of 3 working sets		

CIRCUIT 1

For each circuit, perform the exercises back to back for the specified number of reps. Rest and repeat as indicated.

Push-up	**12** reps	p82
Triceps dip	**12** reps	p86
Medicine ball Russian twist	**16** reps	p54
Rest for 60 seconds		
Repeat twice for a total of 3 rounds		

CIRCUIT 2

Lying dumbbell chest fly	**12** reps	p76
Standing dumbbell shoulder press	**12** reps	p74
Kettlebell windmill (without alternating)	**12** reps/side	p140
Rest for 60 seconds		
Repeat twice for a total of 3 rounds		

CORE FINISHER

Perform the exercises back to back for the specified number of reps. Rest and repeat as indicated.

Side plank warm hug (without alternating)	**10** reps/arm	p52
V-up	**10** reps	p36
High plank shoulder tap (alternating)	**20** reps	p46
Rest for 45 seconds		
Repeat twice for a total of 3 rounds		

DAY 2 Lower body – deadlift

Picking up heavy weights off the ground is one of the best ways to build leg strength. This collection of exercises, including the deadlift, will make your lower body powerful and toned.

MAIN LIFT

Complete 2 warm-up sets with a light resistance. Then do 3 working sets with a challenging resistance (the last 2 reps should be very difficult).

Conventional barbell deadlift (light)	**5** reps	p112
Rest for 60 seconds		
Repeat once for a total of 2 warm-up sets		
Conventional barbell deadlift (heavy)	**8–10** reps	p112
Rest for up to 2 minutes		
Repeat twice for a total of 3 working sets		

SUPERSET

Perform the exercises back to back for the specified number of reps. Rest and repeat as indicated.

Dumbbell reverse lunge (alternating)	**24** reps	p106
Jump lunge	**12** reps	p124
Rest for 45 seconds		
Repeat twice for a total of 3 sets		

CIRCUIT 1

For each circuit, perform the exercises back to back for the specified number of reps or secs. Rest and repeat as indicated.

Dumbbell sumo squat	**12** reps	p94
Single-arm kettlebell clean (alternating)	**20** reps	p134
Forearm plank hold	**30** secs	p45
Rest for 60 seconds		
Repeat twice for a total of 3 rounds		

CIRCUIT 2

Kettlebell single-leg deadlift (without alternating)	**12** reps/leg	p116
Dumbbell lateral lunge (alternating)	**20** reps	p108
Fast mountain climber	**30** secs	p56
Rest for 60 seconds		
Repeat twice for a total of 3 rounds		

DAY 3

Rest

DAY 4 Upper body – pull

Working your back with a barbell effectively builds core and upper-body strength. The medicine ball exercise in the first superset activates your muscle fibres, so you get stronger, faster.

MAIN LIFT

Complete 1 warm-up set with a light resistance. Then do 3 working sets with a challenging resistance (the last 2 reps should be very difficult).		
Barbell bent-over row (light)	**6** reps	p66
Rest for 60 seconds		
Do not repeat warm-up set		
Barbell bent-over row (heavy)	**8–10** reps	p66
Rest for up to 2 minutes		
Repeat twice for a total of 3 working sets		

SUPERSET 1

For each superset, perform the exercises back to back for the specified number of reps. Rest and repeat as indicated.		
Pull-up	**12** reps	p80
Kneeling medicine ball slam	**12** reps	p145
Rest for 60 seconds		
Repeat twice for a total of 3 sets		

SUPERSET 2

Standing dual-dumbbell biceps curl	**12** reps	p88
Dumbbell renegade row (alternating)	**20** reps	p64
Rest for 60 seconds		
Repeat twice for a total of 3 rounds		

CORE FINISHER

Perform the exercises back to back for the specified number of reps. Rest and repeat as indicated.		
Kettlebell plank drag	**10** reps	p48
Side plank hip drop (without alternating)	**12** reps/side	p50
Bicycle crunch	**20** reps	p32
Rest for 45 seconds		
Repeat twice for a total of 3 rounds		

DAY 5 Lower body – squat

These circuits hit your legs with squats, deadlifts, and lunges so that you really feel the burn. The cardio finisher will have you leaving the gym exhausted and satisfied.

MAIN LIFT

Complete 2 warm-up sets with a light resistance. Then do 3 working sets with a challenging resistance (the last 2 reps should be very difficult).		
Barbell back squat (light)	**5** reps	p92
Rest for 60 seconds		
Repeat once for a total of 2 warm-up sets		
Barbell back squat (heavy)	**8–10** reps	p92
Rest for up to 2 minutes		
Repeat twice for a total of 3 working sets		

SUPERSET 1

For each superset, perform the exercises back to back for the specified number of reps. Rest and repeat as indicated.		
Barbell good morning	**12** reps	p100
Dumbbell lateral lunge (alternating)	**20** reps	p108
Rest for 60 seconds		
Repeat twice for a total of 3 sets		

SUPERSET 2

Dumbbell Romanian deadlift	**10** reps	p114
Dumbbell step-up (without alternating)	**10** reps/leg	p110
Rest for 60 seconds		
Repeat twice for a total of 3 rounds		

METABOLIC FINISHER

Perform the exercises back to back for the specified number of reps or secs. Rest and repeat as indicated.		
Box jump	**10** reps	p122
Forearm plank leg march (alternating)	**20** reps	p44
Fast mountain climber	**30** secs	p56
Burpee	**10** reps	p118
Rest for 45 seconds		
Repeat 3 times for a total of 4 rounds		

DAY 6 Rest

DAY 7 Cardio

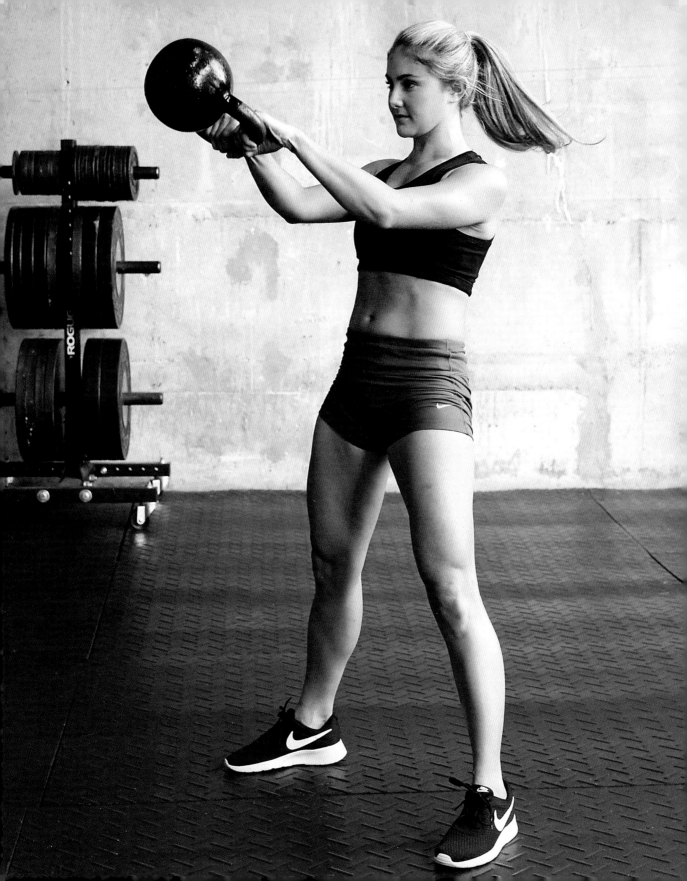

LEVEL 2 Weeks 5–8

The workouts in this phase include more cardio than the first phase, which will help burn fat. The decreased rep ranges help you build more lean muscle mass, but you will need to choose heavier weights during each training session. Follow the weekly schedule, repeating it for a total of 4 consecutive weeks. The workouts are on the following pages. Don't forget to also perform the warm-up and cool-down sequences (pp26–29) on every workout day. After completing all 4 weeks, advance to Level 2: Weeks 9–12.

WEEKLY SCHEDULE	
DAY 1	Upper body – push
DAY 2	Lower body – deadlift
DAY 3	Cardio
DAY 4	Upper body – pull
DAY 5	Lower body – squat
DAY 6	Rest
DAY 7	Cardio

Rest day

You have 1 day to rest during each week of this phase. You can move it around within each week to accommodate your schedule. Push yourself during the workouts so the rest day feels worth it. A rest day is not an inactive day; it's simply a rest day from weights and intense cardio. Take a yoga class or go for a walk, and keep your body moving!

Cardio days

One of your days should be in the form of HIIT, which will blast calories in a short period of time. With a rower or treadmill, alternate between intervals of high-intensity work (sprinting) and low-intensity rest (jogging or walking). Start with a ratio of 30 seconds' work to 60 seconds' rest, and gradually advance to 30 seconds' work to 30 seconds' rest.

For the other day, use cardio equipment or go for a jog outside. Keep the intensity and pace moderate and consistent throughout.

DAY 1 Upper body – push

The first circuit in this workout requires you to use your entire body, not just your arms and shoulders. The remaining circuits hit your arms from every angle.

MAIN LIFT

Complete 2 warm-up sets with a light resistance. Then do 3 working sets with a challenging resistance (the last 2 reps should be very difficult).

Barbell overhead press (light)	**5** reps	p78
Rest for 60 seconds		
Repeat once for a total of 2 warm-up sets		
Barbell overhead press (heavy)	**8–10** reps	p78
Rest for up to 2 minutes		
Repeat twice for a total of 3 working sets		

SUPERSET

Perform the exercises back to back for the specified number of reps. Rest and repeat as indicated.

T push-up (alternating)	**10** reps	p84
V-up	**10** reps	p36
Rest for 45 seconds		
Repeat twice for a total of 3 sets		

CIRCUIT 1

For each circuit, perform the exercises back to back for the specified number of reps or secs. Rest and repeat as indicated.

Standing dumbbell Arnold press	**10** reps	p75
Triceps dip	**10** reps	p86
Kettlebell windmill (without alternating)	**10** reps/side	p140
Rest for 60 seconds		
Repeat twice for a total of 3 rounds		

CIRCUIT 2

Lying dumbbell chest fly	**10** reps	p76
Single-arm kettlebell sit-up (without alternating)	**10** reps/arms	p40
Dumbbell thruster	**30** secs	p146
High plank shoulder tap (alternating)	**20** reps	p46
Rest for 60 seconds		
Repeat twice for a total of 3 rounds		

DAY 2 Lower body – deadlift

Your deadlift reps decrease for these 4 weeks, which means you should be using heavier weights than you did in the last 4 weeks. Challenge yourself for noticeable muscle gains.

MAIN LIFT

Complete 2 warm-up sets with a light resistance. Then do 3 working sets with a challenging resistance (the last 2 reps should be very difficult).

Conventional barbell deadlift (light)	**4** reps	p112
Rest for 60 seconds		
Repeat once for a total of 2 warm-up sets		
Conventional barbell deadlift (heavy)	**6–8** reps	p112
Rest for up to 2 minutes		
Repeat twice for a total of 3 working sets		

SUPERSET

Perform the exercises back to back for the specified number of reps. Rest and repeat as indicated.

Barbell glute bridge	**8** reps	p102
Dumbbell Romanian deadlift	**10** reps	p114
Rest for 45 seconds		
Repeat twice for a total of 3 sets		

CIRCUIT

Perform the exercises back to back for the specified number of reps. Rest and repeat as indicated.

Rear-foot-elevated split squat (without alternating)	**8** reps/side	p98
Dumbbell lateral lunge (alternating)	**20** reps	p108
Jump squat	**10** reps	p128
Rest for 60 seconds		
Repeat twice for a total of 3 rounds		

METABOLIC FINISHER

Perform the exercises back to back for the specified number of reps or secs. Rest and repeat as indicated.

Barbell clean	**8** reps	p136
Russian kettlebell swing	**10** reps	p138
Box jump	**10** reps	p122
Forearm plank hold	**30** secs	p45
Rest for 30 seconds		
Repeat twice for a total of 3 rounds		

DAY 3

Cardio

DAY 4 Upper body – pull

Working your back with a barbell is a great way to build both upper-body and core strength. Remember to perform every rep with perfect technique and control.

MAIN LIFT

Complete 2 warm-up sets with a light resistance. Then do 3 working sets with a challenging resistance (the last 2 reps should be very difficult).

Barbell bent-over row (light)	**6** reps	p66
Rest for 60 seconds		
Repeat once for a total of 2 warm-up sets		
Barbell bent-over row (heavy)	**6–8** reps	p66
Rest for up to 2 minutes		
Repeat twice for a total of 3 working sets		

SUPERSET

Perform the exercises back to back for the specified number of reps. Rest and repeat as indicated.

Staggered stance single-arm row (without alternating)	**8–10** reps/arm	p62
Standing overhead medicine ball slam	**12** reps	p144
Rest for 45 seconds		
Repeat twice for a total of 3 sets		

CIRCUIT 1

For each circuit, perform the exercises back to back for the specified number of reps or steps. Rest and repeat as indicated.

Standing dual-dumbbell biceps curl	**10** reps	p88
Dumbbell upright row	**10** reps	p68
Slow cross mountain climber (alternating)	**20** reps	p58
Rest for 60 seconds		
Repeat twice for a total of 3 rounds		

CIRCUIT 2

Chin-up	**10** reps	p81
Dumbbell renegade row (alternating)	**20** reps	p64
Kettlebell farmer's walk	**30** steps	p60
Burpee	**10** reps	p118
Rest for 60 seconds		
Repeat twice for a total of 3 rounds		

DAY 5 Lower body – squat

As in the last phase, today is all about squats and lunges. This time you will hold the barbell in front of you for the main lift, so you will need to use a lighter resistance.

MAIN LIFT

Complete 2 warm-up sets with a light resistance. Then do 3 working sets with a challenging resistance (the last 2 reps should be very difficult).

Barbell front squat (light)	**5** reps	p90
Rest for 60 seconds		
Repeat once for a total of 2 warm-up sets		
Barbell front squat (heavy)	**6–8** reps	p90
Rest for up to 2 minutes		
Repeat twice for a total of 3 working sets		

CIRCUIT

Perform the exercises back to back for the specified number of reps. Rest and repeat as indicated.

Kettlebell single-leg deadlift (without alternating)	**10** reps/leg	p116
Dumbbell sumo squat	**12** reps	p94
Jump squat	**10** reps	p128
Rest for 60 seconds		
Repeat twice for a total of 3 rounds		

SUPERSET

Perform the exercises back to back for the specified number of reps or steps. Rest and repeat as indicated.

Dumbbell walking lunge	**20** steps	p104
Jump lunge	**20** reps	p124
Rest for 60 seconds		
Repeat twice for a total of 3 sets		

METABOLIC FINISHER

Climb the ladder: perform the exercises back to back, increasing your reps by 2 each round.

Russian kettlebell swing	**2 (4, 6, 8, 10)** reps	p138
Burpee	**2 (4, 6, 8, 10)** reps	p118
Do not rest between rounds		
Repeat 4 times for a total of 5 rounds		

DAY 6 Rest

DAY 7 Cardio

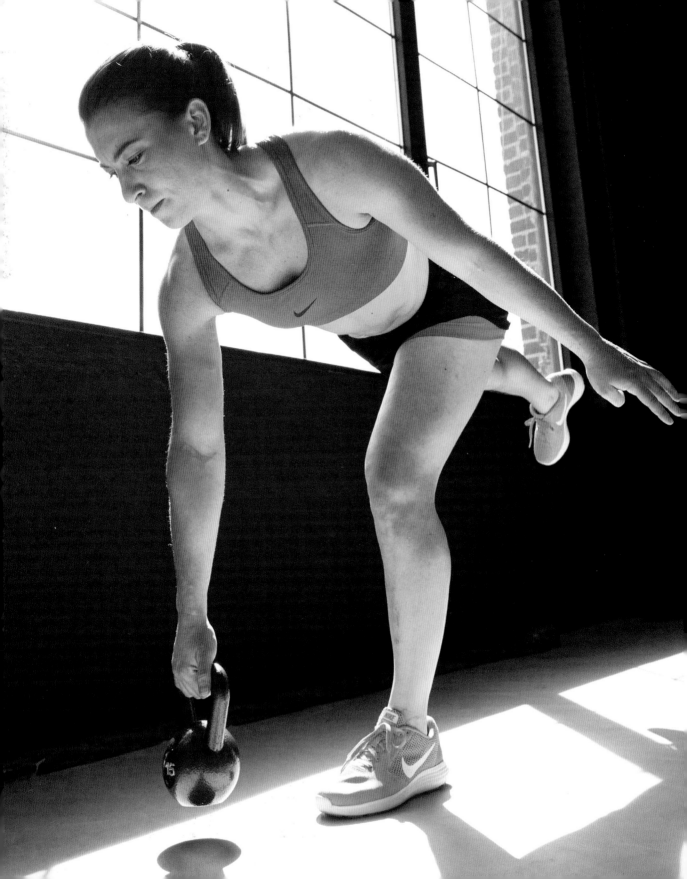

LEVEL 2 Weeks 9–12

In the final phase of Level 2, your main lifts only require 5 reps, so be sure to use the heaviest weight you can manage. However, for all other supersets and circuits, the reps increase to keep your body in a fat-burning state. Follow the weekly schedule, repeating it for a total of 4 consecutive weeks. The workouts are on the following pages. Don't forget to also perform the warm-up and cool-down sequences (pp26–29) on every workout day. After completing all 4 weeks, reassess your fitness and repeat Level 2 or advance to Level 3.

WEEKLY SCHEDULE

DAY 1	Upper body – push
DAY 2	Lower body – deadlift
DAY 3	Cardio
DAY 4	Upper body – pull
DAY 5	Lower body – squat
DAY 6	Rest
DAY 7	Cardio

Rest day
You again have 1 day to rest during each week of this phase. You can move it around within each week to accommodate your schedule. Push yourself during the workouts so the rest day feels worth it. A rest day is not an inactive day; it's simply a rest day from weights and intense cardio. Take a yoga class or go for a walk, and keep your body moving!

Cardio days
One of your days should be in the form of HIIT, which will blast calories in a short period of time. With a rower or treadmill, alternate between intervals of high-intensity work (sprinting) and low-intensity rest (jogging or walking). Start with a ratio of 30 seconds' work to 60 seconds' rest, and gradually advance to 30 seconds' work to 30 seconds' rest. You can also add incline or bodyweight movements to your rest intervals. For example, after every 5 minutes on the machine, hold a 30-second plank or perform 10 bodyweight squats.

For the other day, use cardio equipment or go for a jog outside. Keep the intensity and pace moderate and consistent throughout.

LEVEL 2 Weeks 9–12

DAY 1 Upper body – push

You are only doing 5 reps for the main lift, so go heavier than you have before. Let yourself fully recover between main-lift sets, but keep rest to a minimum for the remainder of the workout.

MAIN LIFT

Complete 2 warm-up sets with a light resistance. Then do 5 working sets with a challenging resistance (the last 2 reps should be very difficult).		
Barbell bench press (light)	**5** reps	p70
Rest for 60 seconds		
Repeat once for a total of 2 warm-up sets		
Barbell bench press (heavy)	**5** reps	p70
Rest for up to 2 minutes		
Repeat 4 times for a total of 5 working sets		

SUPERSET

Perform the exercises back to back for the specified number of reps. Rest and repeat as indicated.		
Barbell push press	**10** reps	p130
Lying dumbbell chest fly	**12** reps	p76
Rest for 45 seconds		
Repeat twice for a total of 3 sets		

CIRCUIT

Perform the exercises back to back for the specified number of reps. Rest and repeat as indicated.		
Standing dual-dumbbell biceps curl	**8** reps	p88
Standing dumbbell Arnold press	**15** reps	p75
Triceps dip	**12** reps	p86
Side plank warm hug (without alternating)	**12** reps/arm	p52
Rest for 60 seconds		
Repeat twice for a total of 3 rounds		

METABOLIC FINISHER

Chipper: perform the exercises back to back, decreasing your reps by 2 each round.		
Russian kettlebell swing	**12 (10, 8, 6, 4, 2)** reps	p138
Standing overhead medicine ball slam	**12 (10, 8, 6, 4, 2)** reps	p144
Burpee	**12 (10, 8, 6, 4, 2)** reps	p118
Do not rest between rounds		
Repeat 5 times for a total of 6 rounds		

DAY 2 Lower body – deadlift

Now that your hinge pattern is perfect, use extremely heavy weights for today's exercises. Your glutes and hamstrings will be burning through every circuit.

MAIN LIFT

Complete 2 warm-up sets with a light resistance. Then do 5 working sets with a challenging resistance (the last 2 reps should be very difficult).		
Conventional barbell deadlift (light)	**3–5** reps	p112
Rest for 60 seconds		
Repeat once for a total of 2 warm-up sets		
Conventional barbell deadlift (heavy)	**5** reps	p112
Rest for up to 2 minutes		
Repeat 4 times for a total of 5 working sets		

CIRCUIT 1

For each circuit, perform the exercises back to back for the specified number of reps or secs. Rest and repeat as indicated.		
Kettlebell single-leg deadlift (without alternating)	**10** reps/leg	p116
Dumbbell lateral lunge (without alternating)	**10** reps/side	p108
Fast mountain climber	**30** secs	p56
Rest for 60 seconds		
Repeat twice for a total of 3 rounds		

CIRCUIT 2

Barbell glute bridge	**15** reps	p102
Dumbbell Romanian deadlift	**15** reps	p114
Jump squat	**30** secs	p128
Rest for 60 seconds		
Repeat twice for a total of 3 rounds		

METABOLIC FINISHER

Chipper: perform the exercises back to back, decreasing your reps by 6 each round.		
Box jump	**15 (9, 3)** reps	p122
Russian kettlebell swing	**15 (9, 3)** reps	p138
Do not rest between rounds		
Repeat twice for a total of 3 rounds		

DAY 3

Cardio

DAY 4 Upper body – pull

This workout challenges your back and shoulder muscles with complex movements. The finisher circuit is the most challenging yet, sure to make you feel athletic and confident.

MAIN LIFT

Complete 2 warm-up sets with a light resistance. Then do 5 working sets with a challenging resistance (the last 2 reps should be very difficult).		
Barbell bent-over row (light)	**5** reps	p66
Rest for 60 seconds		
Repeat once for a total of 2 warm-up sets		
Barbell bent-over row (heavy)	**5** reps	p66
Rest for up to 2 minutes		
Repeat 4 times for a total of 5 working sets		

CIRCUIT 1

For each circuit, perform the exercises back to back for the specified number of reps or secs. Rest and repeat as indicated.		
Pull-up	**15** reps	p80
Standing dual-dumbbell biceps curl	**15** reps	p88
Kettlebell plank drag	**30** secs	p48
Rest for 60 seconds		
Repeat twice for a total of 3 rounds		

CIRCUIT 2

Staggered stance single-arm row (without alternating)	**15** reps/arm	p62
Dual-kettlebell push press	**8** reps	p126
Single-arm dumbbell snatch (without alternating)	**10** reps/side	p132
Rest for 60 seconds		
Repeat twice for a total of 3 rounds		

METABOLIC FINISHER

Perform the exercises back to back for the specified number of reps or secs. Rest and repeat as indicated.		
Dumbbell renegade row (alternating)	**10** reps	p64
Push-up	**10** reps	p82
Fast mountain climber	**30** secs	p56
Burpee	**10** reps	p118
Rest for 45 seconds		
Repeat 3 times for a total of 4 rounds		

DAY 5 Lower body – squat

The low reps mean you can go extraordinarily heavy for the main lift. Exhaust your legs for each circuit, and finish the day with plyometric exercises for huge calorie burn.

MAIN LIFT

Complete 2 warm-up sets with a light resistance. Then do 5 working sets with a challenging resistance (the last 2 reps should be very difficult).		
Barbell back squat (light)	**3–5** reps	p92
Rest for 60 seconds		
Repeat once for a total of 2 warm-up sets		
Barbell back squat (heavy)	**5** reps	p92
Rest for up to 2 minutes		
Repeat 4 times for a total of 5 working sets		

SUPERSET

Perform the exercises back to back for the specified number of reps or secs. Rest and repeat as indicated.		
Rear-foot-elevated split squat (without alternating)	**8** reps/side	p98
Forearm plank hold	**30** secs	p45
Rest for 60 seconds		
Repeat twice for a total of 3 sets		

CIRCUIT 1

For each circuit, perform the exercises back to back for the specified number of reps or steps. Rest and repeat as indicated.		
Dumbbell sumo squat	**10** reps	p94
Dumbbell walking lunge	**12** steps	p104
Butterfly sit-up	**10** reps	p38
Rest for 60 seconds		
Repeat twice for a total of 3 rounds		

CIRCUIT 2

Barbell clean	**8** reps	p136
Russian kettlebell swing	**10** reps	p138
Jump squat	**10** reps	p128
Rest for 60 seconds		
Repeat 3 times for a total of 4 rounds		

METABOLIC FINISHER

5-minute EMOM: using a stopwatch to monitor time, perform the exercises back to back for the specified number of reps, every minute on the minute for 5 minutes total. Rest for the remainder of every minute.		
Box jump	**10** reps	p122
Burpee	**5** reps	p118
Rest until the minute mark		
Repeat for a total of 5 minutes		

DAY 6

Rest

DAY 7

Cardio

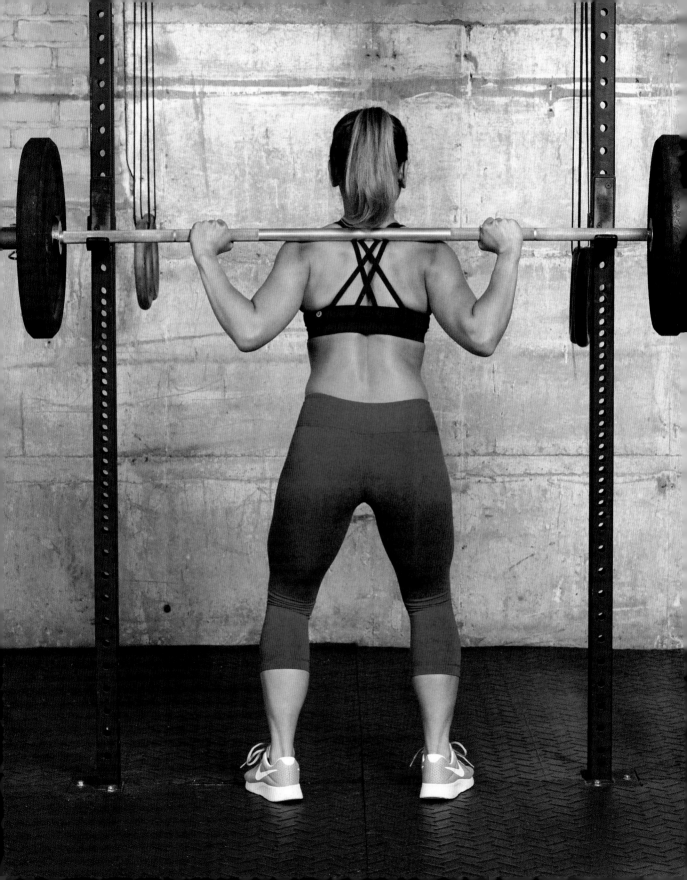

LEVEL 3 Weeks 1-4

With a focus on foundational skills, this first 4-week phase sets you up to lift very heavy weights in the following weeks. Each of your main lifts uses a barbell, so make sure you take adequate rest so you're fresh for each rep. Follow the weekly schedule, repeating it for a total of 4 consecutive weeks. The workouts are on the following pages. Don't forget to also perform the warm-up and cool-down sequences (pp26–29) on every workout day. After completing all 4 weeks, advance to Level 3: Weeks 5–8.

WEEKLY SCHEDULE	
DAY 1	Upper body – push
DAY 2	Lower body – deadlift
DAY 3	Cardio
DAY 4	Upper body – pull
DAY 5	Lower body – squat
DAY 6	Rest
DAY 7	Cardio

Rest day

You have 1 day to rest during each week of this phase. You can move it around within each week to accommodate your schedule. Push yourself during the workouts so the rest day feels worth it. A rest day is not an inactive day; it's simply a rest day from weights and intense cardio. Take a yoga class or go for a walk, and keep your body moving!

Cardio days

One of your days should be in the form of HIIT, which will blast calories in a short period of time. With a rower or treadmill, alternate between intervals of high-intensity work (sprinting) and low-intensity rest (jogging or walking). Start with a ratio of 30 seconds' work to 60 seconds' rest, and gradually advance to 30 seconds' work to 30 seconds' rest. You can also add incline or bodyweight movements to your rest intervals. For example, after every 5 minutes on the machine, hold a 30-second plank or perform 10 bodyweight squats.

For the other day, use cardio equipment or go for a jog outside. Keep the intensity and pace moderate and consistent throughout.

LEVEL 3 Weeks 1–4

DAY 1 Upper body – push

Today's exercises are dedicated to the pushing muscles in your upper body: chest, shoulders, and arms. Move quickly through the supersets for the most effective workout.

MAIN LIFT

Complete 2 warm-up sets with a light resistance. Then do 3 working sets with a challenging resistance (the last 2 reps should be very difficult).

Barbell bench press (light)	5 reps	p70
Rest for 60 seconds		
Repeat once for a total of 2 warm-up sets		
Barbell bench press (heavy)	8–10 reps	p70
Rest for up to 2 minutes		
Repeat twice for a total of 3 working sets		

SUPERSET 1

For each superset, perform the exercises back to back for the specified number of reps. Rest and repeat as indicated.

Declined push-up	5 reps	p83
Medicine ball Russian twist	16 reps	p54
Rest for 45 seconds		
Repeat twice for a total of 3 sets		

SUPERSET 2

Lying dumbbell chest fly	12 reps	p76
Standing dumbbell shoulder press	12 reps	p74
Rest for 45 seconds		
Repeat twice for a total of 3 sets		

SUPERSET 3

Triceps dip	12 reps	p86
Single-arm half-kneeling kettlebell press (without alternating)	10 reps/arm	p72
Rest for 45 seconds		
Repeat twice for a total of 3 sets		

CORE FINISHER

Perform the exercises back to back for the specified number of reps. Rest and repeat as indicated.

Side plank warm hug (without alternating)	12 reps/arm	p52
V-up	15 reps	p36
High plank shoulder tap (alternating)	20 reps	p46
Rest for 30 seconds		
Repeat twice for a total of 3 rounds		

DAY 2 Lower body – deadlift

Start with a deadlift to develop your lower-body strength and power. Then push yourself through the rest of the workout so your glutes, hamstrings, and quads are worn out.

MAIN LIFT

Complete 2 warm-up sets with a light resistance. Then do 3 working sets with a challenging resistance (the last 2 reps should be very difficult).

Conventional barbell deadlift (light)	5 reps	p112
Rest for 60 seconds		
Repeat once for a total of 2 warm-up sets		
Conventional barbell deadlift (heavy)	8–10 reps	p112
Rest for up to 2 minutes		
Repeat twice for a total of 3 working sets		

SUPERSET 1

For each superset, perform the exercises back to back for the specified number of reps. Rest and repeat as indicated.

Dumbbell reverse lunge (alternating)	24 reps	p106
Jump lunge	20 reps	p124
Rest for 45 seconds		
Repeat twice for a total of 3 sets		

SUPERSET 2

Dumbbell sumo squat	24 reps	p94
Single-arm kettlebell clean (without alternating)	10 reps/side	p134
Rest for 45 seconds		
Repeat twice for a total of 3 sets		

CIRCUIT

Perform the exercises back to back for the specified number of reps or secs. Rest and repeat as indicated.

Kettlebell single-leg deadlift (without alternating)	12 reps/leg	p116
Dumbbell lateral lunge (alternating)	20 reps	p108
Fast mountain climber	30 secs	p56
Rest for 30 seconds		
Repeat twice for a total of 3 rounds		

DAY 3 Cardio

DAY 4 Upper body – pull

This workout challenges your upper-body pulling muscles. Finish the day with a core circuit to further tone your physique and make all your movements more stable.

MAIN LIFT

Complete 1 warm-up set with a light resistance. Then do 3 working sets with a challenging resistance (the last 2 reps should be very difficult).		
Barbell bent-over row (light)	**6** reps	p66
Rest for 60 seconds		
Do not repeat warm-up set		
Barbell bent-over row (heavy)	**10–12** reps	p66
Rest for up to 2 minutes		
Repeat twice for a total of 3 working sets		

SUPERSET 1

For each superset, perform the exercises back to back for the specified number of reps. Rest and repeat as indicated.		
Pull-up	**12** reps	p80
Kneeling medicine ball slam	**12** reps	p145
Rest for 45 seconds		
Repeat twice for a total of 3 sets		

SUPERSET 2

Standing dual-dumbbell biceps curl	**12** reps	p88
Dumbbell renegade row (alternating)	**24** reps	p64
Rest for 45 seconds		
Repeat twice for a total of 3 sets		

SUPERSET 3

Staggered stance single-arm row (without alternating)	**12** reps/arm	p62
Dumbbell upright row	**12** reps	p68
Rest for 45 seconds		
Repeat twice for a total of 3 sets		

CORE FINISHER

Perform the exercises back to back for the specified number of reps. Rest and repeat as indicated.		
Kettlebell plank drag	**10** reps	p48
Side plank hip drop (without alternating)	**12** reps/side	p50
Bicycle crunch	**20** reps	p32
Rest for 30 seconds		
Repeat twice for a total of 3 rounds		

DAY 5 Lower body – squat

Today's lower-body workout will fire up your entire posterior chain – the back side of the body – while also developing overall leg power and strength.

MAIN LIFT

Complete 2 warm-up sets with a light resistance. Then do 3 working sets with a challenging resistance (the last 2 reps should be very difficult).		
Barbell back squat (light)	**5** reps	p92
Rest for 60 seconds		
Repeat once for a total of 2 warm-up sets		
Barbell back squat (heavy)	**8–10** reps	p92
Rest for up to 2 minutes		
Repeat twice for a total of 3 working sets		

SUPERSET

Perform the exercises back to back for the specified number of reps. Rest and repeat as indicated.		
Barbell good morning	**12** reps	p100
Dumbbell lateral lunge (alternating)	**20** reps	p108
Rest for 45 seconds		
Repeat twice for a total of 3 sets		

CIRCUIT

Perform the exercises back to back for the specified number of reps. Rest and repeat as indicated.		
Dumbbell Romanian deadlift	**12** reps	p114
Dumbbell step-up (without alternating)	**10** reps/leg	p110
Russian kettlebell swing	**10** reps	p138
Rest for 60 seconds		
Repeat twice for a total of 3 rounds		

CORE FINISHER

Perform the exercises back to back for the specified number of reps or secs. Rest and repeat as indicated.		
Forearm plank leg march (alternating)	**20** reps	p44
Fast mountain climber	**30** secs	p56
Burpee	**10** reps	p118
Rest for 30 seconds		
Repeat 3 times for a total of 4 rounds		

DAY 6 DAY 7

Rest Cardio

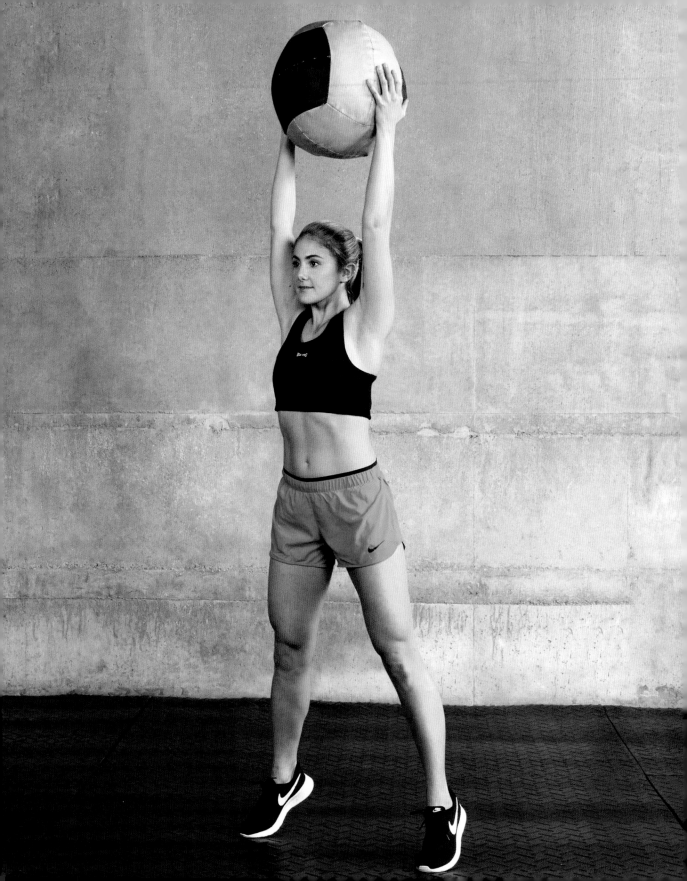

LEVEL 3 Weeks 5–8

For this second phase, you will burn fat and build muscle with heavy resistance and conditioning circuits. Push yourself hard during the cardio circuits to make each training session worthwhile. Follow the weekly schedule, repeating it for a total of 4 consecutive weeks. The workouts are on the following pages. Don't forget to also perform the warm-up and cool-down sequences (pp26–29) on every workout day. After completing all 4 weeks, advance to Level 3: Weeks 9–12.

WEEKLY SCHEDULE	
DAY 1	Upper body – push
DAY 2	Lower body – deadlift
DAY 3	Cardio
DAY 4	Upper body – pull
DAY 5	Lower body – squat
DAY 6	Rest
DAY 7	Cardio

Rest day

You again have 1 day to rest during each week of this phase. You can move it around within each week to accommodate your schedule. Push yourself during the workouts so the rest day feels worth it. A rest day is not an inactive day; it's simply a rest day from weights and intense cardio. Take a yoga class or go for a walk, and keep your body moving!

Cardio days

One of your days should be in the form of HIIT, which will blast calories in a short period of time. With a rower or treadmill, alternate between intervals of high-intensity work (sprinting) and low-intensity rest (jogging or walking). Start with a ratio of 30 seconds' work to 60 seconds' rest, and gradually advance to 30 seconds' work to 30 seconds' rest. You can also add incline or bodyweight movements to your rest intervals. For example, after every 5 minutes on the machine, hold a 30-second plank or perform 10 bodyweight squats.

For the other day, use cardio equipment or go for a jog outside. Keep the intensity and pace moderate and consistent throughout.

LEVEL 3 Weeks 5–8

DAY 1 Upper body – push

Today's focus is your shoulders for the main lift – the overhead press. Engage your entire body while pressing the barbell up, and keep up the intensity for the remaining workout.

MAIN LIFT

Complete 1 warm-up set with a light resistance. Then do 3 working sets with a challenging resistance (the last 2 reps should be very difficult).		
Barbell overhead press (light)	**6** reps	p78
Rest for 60 seconds		
Do not repeat warm-up set		
Barbell overhead press (heavy)	**8–10** reps	p78
Rest for up to 2 minutes		
Repeat twice for a total of 3 working sets		

SUPERSET

Perform the exercises back to back for the specified number of reps. Rest and repeat as indicated.		
Plyo push-up	**8–10** reps	p120
V-up	**10** reps	p36
Rest for 45 seconds		
Repeat twice for a total of 3 sets		

CIRCUIT 1

For each circuit, perform the exercises back to back for the specified number of reps. Rest and repeat as indicated.		
Triceps dip	**10** reps	p86
Kettlebell windmill (without alternating)	**8–10** reps/side	p140
Kneeling ring rollout	**10** reps	p42
Rest for 45 seconds		
Repeat twice for a total of 3 rounds		

CIRCUIT 2

Lying dumbbell chest fly	**10** reps	p76
Dumbbell upright row	**10** reps	p68
Single-arm dumbbell snatch (without alternating)	**10** reps/side	p132
Rest for 45 seconds		
Repeat twice for a total of 3 rounds		

CIRCUIT 3

Dual-kettlebell push press	**10** reps	p126
Side plank warm hug (without alternating)	**10** reps/arm	p52
High plank shoulder tap (alternating)	**20** reps	p46
Rest for 30 seconds		
Repeat twice for a total of 3 rounds		

DAY 2 Lower body – deadlift

Your deadlift reps drop for this workout compared to previous weeks, so load the barbell with exceptionally heavy weights. Push yourself with the same intensity for every circuit to see results.

MAIN LIFT

Complete 2 warm-up sets with a light resistance. Then do 3 working sets with challenging resistance (the last 2 reps should be very difficult).		
Conventional barbell deadlift (light)	**4** reps	p112
Rest for 60 seconds		
Repeat once for a total of 2 warm-up sets		
Conventional barbell deadlift (heavy)	**6–8** reps	p112
Rest for up to 2 minutes		
Repeat twice for a total of 3 working sets		

CIRCUIT 1

For each circuit, perform the exercises back to back for the specified number of reps or secs. Rest and repeat as indicated.		
Barbell glute bridge	**8** reps	p102
Dumbbell lateral lunge (alternating)	**16** reps	p108
Forearm plank leg march (alternating)	**20** reps	p44
Rest for 45 seconds		
Repeat twice for a total of 3 rounds		

CIRCUIT 2

Rear-foot-elevated split squat (without alternating)	**8** reps/side	p98
Jump squat	**10** reps	p128
Forearm plank hold	**30** secs	p45
Rest for 45 seconds		
Repeat twice for a total of 3 rounds		

METABOLIC FINISHER

Perform the exercises back to back for the specified number of reps. Rest and repeat as indicated.		
Barbell clean	**8** reps	p136
Russian kettlebell swing	**10** reps	p138
Box jump	**10** reps	p122
Rest for 30 seconds		
Repeat 3 times for a total of 4 rounds		

DAY 3 Cardio

DAY 4 Upper body – pull

Your shoulders are important for both pushing and pulling movements, but today's main lift and supersets focus particularly on their pulling and stabilizing capabilities.

MAIN LIFT

Complete 2 warm-up sets with a light resistance. Then do 3 working sets with a challenging resistance (the last 2 reps should be very difficult).		
Barbell bent-over row (light)	**6** reps	p66
Rest for 60 seconds		
Repeat once for a total of 2 warm-up sets		
Barbell bent-over row (heavy)	**8–10** reps	p66
Rest for up to 2 minutes		
Repeat twice for a total of 3 working sets		

SUPERSET 1

For each superset, perform the exercises back to back for the specified number of reps. Rest and repeat as indicated.		
Staggered stance single-arm row (without alternating)	**8–10** reps/arm	p62
Standing overhead medicine ball slam	**12** reps	p144
Rest for 45 seconds		
Repeat twice for a total of 3 sets		

SUPERSET 2

Standing dual-dumbbell biceps curl	**10** reps	p88
Slow cross mountain climber (alternating)	**20** reps	p58
Rest for 45 seconds		
Repeat twice for a total of 3 sets		

SUPERSET 3

Dumbbell upright row	**10** reps	p68
Dumbbell renegade row (alternating)	**20** reps	p64
Rest for 45 seconds		
Repeat twice for a total of 3 sets		

CIRCUIT

Perform the exercises back to back for the specified number of reps. Rest and repeat as indicated.		
Chin-up	**10** reps	p81
Kettlebell plank drag	**20** reps	p48
Burpee	**10** reps	p118
Rest for 30 seconds		
Repeat 3 times for a total of 4 rounds		

DAY 5 Lower body – squat

Use perfect form for your lunges, and go a little deeper into your squats to make today's workout worthwhile. Use heavy weights so that every rep is challenging and uncomfortable.

MAIN LIFT

Complete 2 warm-up sets with a light resistance. Then do 3 working sets with a challenging resistance (the last 2 reps should be very difficult).		
Barbell front squat (light)	**6** reps	p90
Rest for 60 seconds		
Repeat once for a total of 2 warm-up sets		
Barbell front squat (heavy)	**8–10** reps	p90
Rest for up to 2 minutes		
Repeat twice for a total of 3 working sets		

SUPERSET 1

For each superset, perform the exercises back to back for the specified number of reps or steps. Rest and repeat as indicated.		
Kettlebell single-leg deadlift (without alternating)	**10** reps/leg	p116
Dumbbell Romanian deadlift	**10** reps	p114
Rest for 45 seconds		
Repeat twice for a total of 3 sets		

SUPERSET 2

Dumbbell walking lunge	**20** steps	p104
Jump lunge	**20** reps	p124
Rest for 45 seconds		
Repeat twice for a total of 3 sets		

SUPERSET 3

Dumbbell sumo squat	**12** reps	p94
Jump squat	**10** reps	p128
Rest for 45 seconds		
Repeat twice for a total of 3 sets		

METABOLIC FINISHER

Climb the ladder: perform the exercises back to back, increasing your reps by 2 each round.		
Barbell thruster	**2 (4, 6, 8, 10)** reps	p148
Box jump	**2 (4, 6, 8, 10)** reps	p122
Do not rest between sets		
Repeat 4 times for a total of 5 sets		

DAY 6
Rest

DAY 7
Cardio

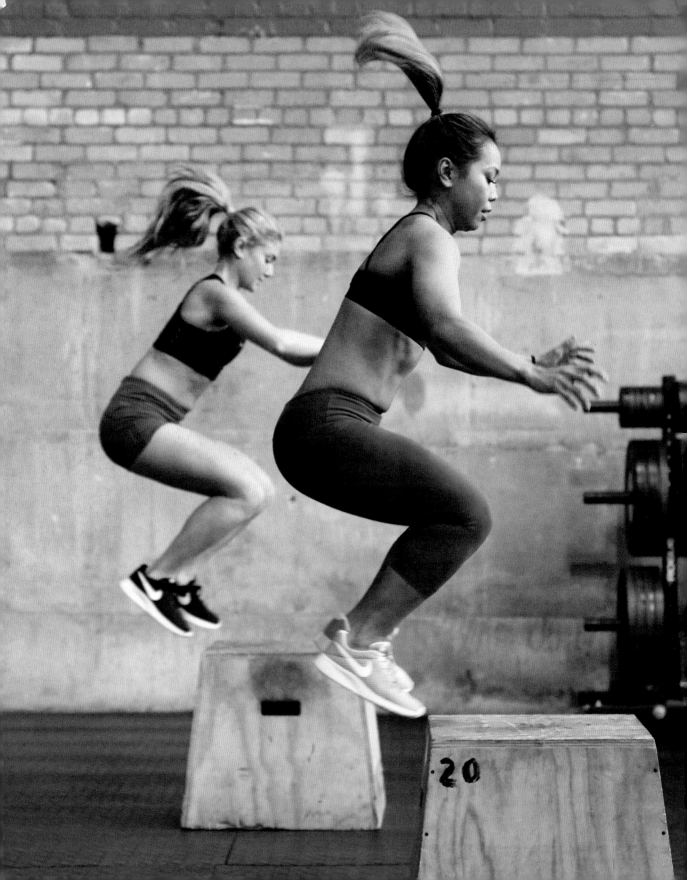

LEVEL 3 Weeks 9–12

These 4 weeks have everything – complex power lifts, tough cardio circuits, and isolation exercises to define your muscles. You made it to the last phase of a very advanced programme, so be proud of yourself, and don't let your intensity falter. Follow the weekly schedule, repeating it for a total of 4 consecutive weeks. The workouts are on the following pages. Don't forget to also perform the warm-up and cool-down sequences (pp26–29) on every workout day. After completing all 4 weeks, repeat Level 3 using heavier weights and doing harder variations of exercises.

WEEKLY SCHEDULE

DAY 1	Upper body – push
DAY 2	Lower body – deadlift
DAY 3	Cardio
DAY 4	Upper body – pull
DAY 5	Lower body – squat
DAY 6	Rest
DAY 7	Cardio

Rest day
You still have 1 day to rest during each week of this phase. You can move it around within each week to accommodate your schedule. Push yourself during the workouts so the rest day feels worth it. A rest day is not an inactive day; it's simply a rest day from weights and intense cardio. Take a yoga class or go for a walk, and keep your body moving!

Cardio days
One of your days should be in the form of HIIT, which will blast calories in a short period of time. With a rower or treadmill, alternate between intervals of high-intensity work (sprinting) and low-intensity rest (jogging or walking). Start with a ratio of 30 seconds' work to 60 seconds' rest, and gradually advance to 30 seconds' work to 30 seconds' rest. You can also add incline or bodyweight movements to your rest intervals. For example, after every 5 minutes on the machine, hold a 30-second plank or perform 10 bodyweight squats.

For the other day, use cardio equipment or go for a jog outside. Keep the intensity and pace moderate and consistent throughout.

LEVEL 3 Weeks 9–12

DAY 1 Upper body – push

Today's barbell press and kettlebell clean will make you feel exceptionally strong and capable. The tabata finishers will help you burn fat fast and make your heart rate skyrocket.

MAIN LIFT

Complete 2 warm-up sets with a light resistance. Then do 3 working sets with a challenging resistance (the last 2 reps should be very difficult).		
Barbell bench press (light)	**5** reps	p70
Rest for 60 seconds		
Repeat once for a total of 2 warm-up sets		
Barbell bench press (heavy)	**5** reps	p70
Rest for up to 2 minutes		
Repeat twice for a total of 3 working sets		

CIRCUIT 1

For each circuit, perform the exercises back to back for the specified number of reps. Rest and repeat as indicated.		
Barbell push press	**15** reps	p130
Dumbbell upright row	**15** reps	p68
Lying dumbbell chest fly	**12** reps	p76
Rest for 45 seconds		
Repeat twice for a total of 3 sets		

CIRCUIT 2

Dumbbell renegade row (alternating)	**16** reps	p64
Single-arm kettlebell clean (without alternating)	**10** reps/ side	p134
Side plank warm hug (without alternating)	**10** reps/ arm	p52
Rest for 45 seconds		
Repeat twice for a total of 3 rounds		

CIRCUIT 3

Standing dumbbell Arnold press	**15** reps	p75
Plyo push-up	**10** reps	p120
Kettlebell plank drag	**20** reps	p48
Rest for 45 seconds		
Repeat twice for a total of 3 rounds		

METABOLIC FINISHER

Tabata: perform the exercises back to back with 10 seconds of rest between each round for a total of 4 minutes (8 rounds).		
Wall ball	**20** secs	p142
V-up	**20** secs	p36
Rest for 10 seconds		
Repeat for a total of 4 minutes		

DAY 2 Lower body – deadlift

This workout is all about your glutes. They are a big muscle group, so go hard on them. The finisher involves working hard without rest, so you'll be burning calories long after you're done.

MAIN LIFT

Complete 2 warm-up sets with a light resistance. Then do 5 working sets with a challenging resistance (the last 2 reps should be very difficult).		
Conventional barbell deadlift (light)	**3–5** reps	p112
Rest for 60 seconds		
Repeat once for a total of 2 warm-up sets		
Conventional barbell deadlift (heavy)	**5** reps	p112
Rest for up to 2 minutes		
Repeat 4 times for a total of 5 working sets		

CIRCUIT 1

For each circuit, perform the exercises back to back for the specified number of reps or secs. Rest and repeat as indicated.		
Rear-foot-elevated split squat (without alternating)	**10** reps/ side	p98
Dumbbell lateral lunge (without alternating)	**12** reps/ side	p108
Fast mountain climber	**30** secs	p56
Rest for 45 seconds		
Repeat twice for a total of 3 rounds		

CIRCUIT 2

Kettlebell single-leg deadlift (without alternating)	**13** reps/ leg	p116
Barbell glute bridge	**15** reps	p102
Dumbbell Romanian deadlift	**15** reps	p114
Jump squat	**30** secs	p128
Rest for 45 seconds		
Repeat twice for a total of 3 rounds		

METABOLIC FINISHER

Chipper: perform the exercises back to back, decreasing your reps by 6 each round.		
Box jump	**21 (15, 9)** reps	p122
Russian kettlebell swing	**21 (15, 9)** reps	p138
Do not rest between rounds		
Repeat twice for a total of 3 rounds		

DAY 3

Cardio

DAY 4 Upper body – pull

For today's main lift, focus on proper form and smooth, controlled movements. Challenge yourself, but don't go so heavy that you risk improper technique or injury.

MAIN LIFT

Complete 2 warm-up sets with a light resistance. Then do 5 working sets with a challenging resistance (the last 2 reps should be very difficult).

Barbell bent-over row (light)	**5** reps	p66
Rest for 60 seconds		
Repeat once for a total of 2 warm-up sets		
Barbell bent-over row (heavy)	**5** reps	p66
Rest for up to 2 minutes		
Repeat 4 times for a total of 5 working sets		

CIRCUIT 1

For each circuit, perform the exercises back to back for the specified number of reps. Rest and repeat as indicated.

Staggered stance single-arm row (without alternating)	**15** reps/arm	p62
Standing overhead medicine ball slam	**12** reps	p144
Side plank hip drop (without alternating)	**10** reps/side	p50
Rest for 45 seconds		
Repeat twice for a total of 3 rounds		

CIRCUIT 2

Dual-kettlebell push press	**15** reps	p126
Single-arm dumbbell snatch (without alternating)	**10** reps/side	p132
Kneeling ring rollout	**12** reps	p42
Rest for 45 seconds		
Repeat twice for a total of 3 rounds		

METABOLIC FINISHER

Perform the exercises back to back for the specified number of reps. Rest and repeat as indicated.

Dumbbell renegade row (alternating)	**20** reps	p64
Pull-up	**10** reps	p80
Plyo push-up	**10** reps	p120
Burpee	**10** reps	p118
Rest for 30 seconds		
Repeat 4 times for a total of 5 rounds		

DAY 5 Lower body – squat

Since it's your final day of the programme, work harder and with heavier weights than you have before. Your 3 conditioning circuits will improve leg and hip power while torching calories.

MAIN LIFT

Complete 2 warm-up sets with a light resistance . Then do 5 working sets with a challenging resistance (the last 2 reps should be very difficult).

Barbell back squat (light)	**3–5** reps	p92
Rest for 60 seconds		
Repeat once for a total of 2 warm-up sets		
Barbell back squat (heavy)	**5** reps	p92
Rest for up to 2 minutes		
Repeat 4 times for a total of 5 working sets		

CIRCUIT 1

For each circuit, perform the exercises back to back for the specified number of reps, secs, or steps. Rest and repeat as indicated.

Rear-foot-elevated split squat (without alternating)	**8** reps/side	p98
V-up	**10** reps	p36
Forearm plank hold	**30** secs	p45
Rest for 45 seconds		
Repeat twice for a total of 3 rounds		

CIRCUIT 2

Dumbbell sumo squat	**10** reps	p94
Dumbbell walking lunge	**20** steps	p104
Slow cross mountain climber (alternating)	**20** reps	p58
Rest for 45 seconds		
Repeat twice for a total of 3 rounds		

CIRCUIT 3

Barbell clean	**8** reps	p136
Russian kettlebell swing	**10** reps	p138
Jump squat	**10** reps	p128
Rest for 45 seconds		
Repeat 3 times for a total of 4 rounds		

METABOLIC FINISHER

6-minute EMOM: using a stopwatch to monitor time, perform the exercises back to back for the specified number of reps, every minute on the minute for 6 minutes total. Rest for the remainder of every minute.

Dumbbell thruster	**10** reps	p146
Burpee	**6** reps	p118
Rest until the minute mark		
Repeat for a total of 6 minutes		

DAY 6 Rest

DAY 7 Cardio

INDEX

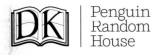
Penguin Random House

DK UK
Senior editor Kate Meeker
Senior art editor Glenda Fisher
Angliciser Kate Berens
Jacket designers Harriet Yeomans and Steven Marsden
Creative technical support Sonia Charbonnier
Pre-production producer Rebecca Fallowfield
Producer Luca Bazzoli
Managing editor Stephanie Farrow
Managing art editor Christine Keilty

DK US
Editor Alexandra Elliott
Senior editor Ann Barton
Book designer Mandy Earey
Art director for photography Nigel Wright
Photographer Jason Riker
Associate publisher Billy Fields
Publisher Mike Sanders

First published in Great Britain in 2018 by
Dorling Kindersley Limited
80 Strand, London, WC2R 0RL

A CIP catalogue record for this book
is available from the British Library.
ISBN: 978–0–2413–0589–8

Printed and bound in China.

All images © Dorling Kindersley Limited
For further information see: www.dkimages.com

A WORLD OF IDEAS:
SEE ALL THERE IS TO KNOW

www.dk.com

ABOUT THE AUTHOR

Alex Silver-Fagan discovered her love for fitness and lifting weights while at university. She felt strong and unstoppable when in the gym, a feeling she had not experienced before. After graduating from New York University, Alex began to explore a variety of fitness styles, both professionally and personally – from bodybuilding and bikini competitions, all the way to CrossFit and group fitness.

Now Alex is an ACE-certified personal trainer, a group fitness instructor, a 200-hour certified yoga teacher, a sponsored athlete on TEAM Bodybuilding.com, and holds multiple certifications, including: KBA 1 kettlebell, FMS, and CFSC. She began teaching classes and training private clients in 2015, and she was soon chosen by NIKE as one of their top NYC trainers.

Alex's fitness methodology emphasizes balance, nutrition, cardio performance, and resistance training, all with the underlying goal of achieving confidence and strength.

AUTHOR'S THANKS

First and foremost, I dedicate this book to you and your fitness journey. You've already taken the first step, now simply stay focused, have patience, and crush it!

Thank you to my dad for always encouraging me to chase my dreams, and thank you to my grandma for your endless love and support.

Big shout out to everyone at Solace New York, my home gym and my family.

Thank you to Ann Barton and Alexandra Elliott at DK for making this first authoring experience simple, fun, and exciting. Also, special thanks to Nigel Wright, Jason Riker, and Christie Caiola for their amazing job on all of the photos, and to my gorgeous and strong models (Carla, Kristie, Natalia, and Sami) for bringing the vision to life.

PUBLISHER'S ACKNOWLEDGMENTS

DK would like to thank the following:

Models Sami Chheng, Carla Miranda, Kristie Muller, Natalia Roberts, and Alex Silver-Fagan

Makeup artist and hair stylist Christie Caiola

Proofreader Laura Caddell

Indexer Brad Herriman